SpringerBriefs in Statistics

SpringerBriefs present concise summaries of cutting-edge research and practical applications across a wide spectrum of fields. Featuring compact volumes of 50 to 125 pages, the series covers a range of content from professional to academic. Typical topics might include:

- A timely report of state-of-the art analytical techniques
- A bridge between new research results, as published in journal articles, and a contextual literature review
- A snapshot of a hot or emerging topic
- An in-depth case study or clinical example
- A presentation of core concepts that students must understand in order to make independent contributions

SpringerBriefs in Statistics showcase emerging theory, empirical research, and practical application in Statistics from a global author community.

SpringerBriefs are characterized by fast, global electronic dissemination, standard publishing contracts, standardized manuscript preparation and formatting guidelines, and expedited production schedules.

Edward Gunning • John Warmenhoven •
Andrew J. Harrison • Norma Bargary

Functional Data Analysis in Biomechanics

A Concise Review of Core Techniques, Applications and Emerging Areas

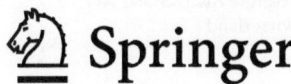 Springer

Edward Gunning
Department of Biostatistics, Epidemiology
and Informatics
University of Pennsylvania
Philadelphia, PA, USA

Andrew J. Harrison
Department of Physical Education and
Sport Sciences
University of Limerick
Limerick, Ireland

John Warmenhoven
School of Sport, Exercise and Rehabilitation
University of Technology Sydney
Sydney, NSW, Australia

Norma Bargary
MACSI, Department of Mathematics and
Statistics
University of Limerick
Limerick, Ireland

ISSN 2191-544X   ISSN 2191-5458   (electronic)
SpringerBriefs in Statistics
ISBN 978-3-031-68861-4   ISBN 978-3-031-68862-1   (eBook)
https://doi.org/10.1007/978-3-031-68862-1

© The Author(s), under exclusive license to Springer Nature Switzerland AG 2024

This work is subject to copyright. All rights are solely and exclusively licensed by the Publisher, whether the whole or part of the material is concerned, specifically the rights of translation, reprinting, reuse of illustrations, recitation, broadcasting, reproduction on microfilms or in any other physical way, and transmission or information storage and retrieval, electronic adaptation, computer software, or by similar or dissimilar methodology now known or hereafter developed.
The use of general descriptive names, registered names, trademarks, service marks, etc. in this publication does not imply, even in the absence of a specific statement, that such names are exempt from the relevant protective laws and regulations and therefore free for general use.
The publisher, the authors and the editors are safe to assume that the advice and information in this book are believed to be true and accurate at the date of publication. Neither the publisher nor the authors or the editors give a warranty, expressed or implied, with respect to the material contained herein or for any errors or omissions that may have been made. The publisher remains neutral with regard to jurisdictional claims in published maps and institutional affiliations.

This Springer imprint is published by the registered company Springer Nature Switzerland AG
The registered company address is: Gewerbestrasse 11, 6330 Cham, Switzerland

If disposing of this product, please recycle the paper.

Preface

As technology advances rapidly and data collection becomes more complex, our ability to capture and record good quality, high-frequency data from biomechanical systems has grown exponentially. This presents an opportunity to gain deeper insights into the complexities of human movement, and a challenge to provide the tools required to most effectively analyse and interpret the resulting data.

Functional data analysis (FDA) and human movement have been intrinsically linked since the seminal work of Ramsay [1], Rice and Silverman [2] and Leurgans et al. [3]. FDA provides a powerful statistical framework for unlocking insights from modern biomechanical data, allowing us to model entire sequences of measurements as single functional entities, and provide new opportunities to improve understanding of movement dynamics. Although FDA has enjoyed growing popularity within the biomechanics community, analyses have typically focused on the use of functional principal component analysis (FPCA). While FPCA is often useful and forms a key component in many of the more complex FDA procedures, it is not the appropriate approach to use in all settings. Additionally, the theoretical focus of much FDA work, and the lack of resources available that outline the full suite of FDA methods available to address challenges encountered in biomechanics and human movement research, has contributed to a lower uptake of FDA in these research communities than might be anticipated despite its clear advantages.

Our aim with this book is to bridge that gap, providing a valuable resource for biomechanics researchers seeking to broaden or deepen their FDA knowledge. While we draw on previous work, particularly that of Ramsay and Silverman [4], we provide an applications-focused approach using open source biomechanical datasets (GaitRec [5], children's gait data [6] and juggling data [7, 8]). Therefore, we hope that this text acts as both a contextual literature review of FDA applications in biomechanics and an introduction to FDA techniques for applied researchers. We also provide an R code repository to carry out the associated analyses for each chapter. This can be found on GitHub at https://github.com/FAST-ULxNUIG/SpringerBriefs.

We believe the content of this book will appeal to all sectors of biomechanics as well as practitioners in other related fields of research where data present in the form of time series or curves. We hope you enjoy your journey through Functional Data Analysis in Biomechanics!

Philadelphia, PA, USA   Dr Edward Gunning
Limerick, Ireland   Professor Drew Harrison
Sydney, NSW, Australia   Dr John Warmenhoven
Limerick, Ireland   Professor Norma Bargary

Acknowledgements

This book has emanated from research conducted with the financial support of Science Foundation Ireland under Grant numbers 18/CRT/6049 (Dr Edward Gunning) and 19/FFP/7002 (Prof. Norma Bargary). We would also like to acknowledge the contributions of numerous colleagues and collaborators who have provided invaluable input to the author team.

Contents

Chapter 1
Introduction

Abstract This introductory chapter summarises the characteristics of modern biomechanical data which have motivated the use of functional data analysis techniques in biomechanics and human movement science. It introduces the main ideas in functional data analysis (FDA) and gives a brief history of the long-standing link between FDA and applications to human movement biomechanics. It then summarises the recent growing popularity of FDA methods in the field, and highlights how developments in FDA methodology have scope for wider uptake and application in biomechanics.

Keywords Functional data analysis · Biomechanics · Big data

1.1 "Big Data" in Biomechanics

Over the last two decades, the field of *human movement biomechanics*, which Winter [9, p. 1] defines as "the inter-discipline that describes, analyses, and assesses human movement", has undergone a "big data" revolution. Improvements in existing technologies (e.g., motion capture equipment) and the introduction of new technologies (e.g., wearable sensors) have led to a proliferation of data that can be used to improve understanding of sports performance, healthy and impaired movement and the effects of treatments and therapies [5, 10–14]. Twentieth-century biomechanics research generally involved a small number of subjects and variables, limited by processing demands on the data produced [10], and relied on hypothesis testing with parametric statistical tests [14, p. 2]. However, characteristics of modern biomechanical data and the demand for greater depth of analysis make these approaches unsuitable or inefficient. For example, motion capture data can now be recorded, processed and extracted efficiently for each subject, meaning that data from a single movement can comprise thousands or hundreds of thousands of measurements [11]. Wearable sensor technologies now offer a viable alternative to these systems, enabling the collection of rich biomechanical datasets outside of traditional laboratory environments [15]. In many instances, the number of subjects in biomechanical datasets is still small (e.g., between 10 and 50; see

© The Author(s), under exclusive license to Springer Nature Switzerland AG 2024
E. Gunning et al., *Functional Data Analysis in Biomechanics*,
SpringerBriefs in Statistics, https://doi.org/10.1007/978-3-031-68862-1_1

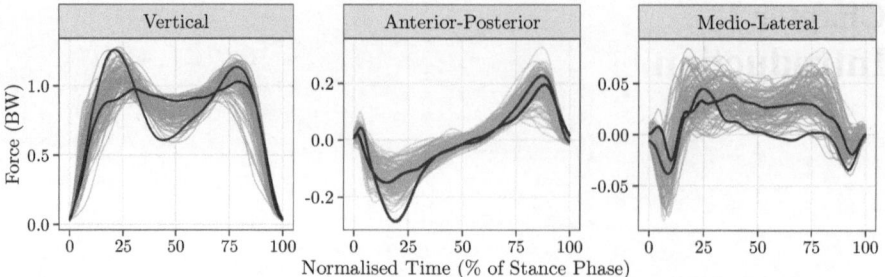

Fig. 1.1 A sample of data from the GaitRec dataset. The grey lines display measurements of the vertical, anterior-posterior and medio-lateral ground reaction force (GRF) components during the stance phase of walking for a random sample of 100 walking trials. Two walking trials from different individuals are highlighted in blue and red, respectively. **Note**: The full dataset is publicly available at https://doi.org/10.6084/m9.figshare.c.4788012.v1

Phinyomark et al. [10]), but some large, open-source datasets such as GaitRec [5], which contains data on walking trials of 2295 individuals under different conditions (75,732 trials in total), have been released (Fig. 1.1). Movement data need to be linked to other information such as sports performance variables, the presence of pathologies, anthropometric measurements, and complex hierarchical structures. They can also be noisy, incomplete or irregularly sampled for various reasons [10, 11, 14]. To deal with and leverage the rich and complex structures of modern biomechanical datasets, researchers have started to employ modern techniques from machine learning and high-dimensional statistics. Among these, functional data analysis (FDA) has emerged as a very natural framework for modelling the high-dimensional, time-dependent data that are collected, as it assumes they arise from a smooth, time-varying function [11, 16, 17].

1.2 Functional Data Analysis

FDA is a sub-field of statistics concerned with the processing, description, analysis and interpretation of data that can be described as smooth functions (e.g., curves, surfaces, or images). FDA was established as an area of research in the 1980s through contributions by Ramsay [1] and Besse and Ramsay [18], who extended classical multivariate statistical techniques, where observations present as vectors, to the setting where observations are smooth functions. Theoretical and method-ological developments and innovative applications of FDA in diverse fields surged in the late 1990's and 2000's. These advances were due, in part, to a seminal textbook by Ramsay and Silverman [4] (first edition published in 1997), improved computing resources and the availability of bespoke FDA software [19, 20], and advancements in recording, processing and storage technologies facilitating the widespread collection of data varying over time, space and other continua.

In the traditional FDA setting, functional data comprise a sample of N real-valued curves, denoted by $x_1(t), \ldots, x_N(t)$, which are defined on an interval $[0, T]$ [21]; most commonly, this interval represents time. Unlike the vectors containing fixed numbers of variables that are encountered in multivariate statistics, functions are infinite-dimensional objects because they are defined at every $t \in [0, T]$. In practice, functional data are typically measured (or sampled) at discrete points, so they often present as very high-dimensional vectors. In this setting, the natural ordering of the measurements and the belief that a smooth function underlies them distinguishes the FDA philosophy from the classical multivariate case [4, 22–24]. Wang et al. [21] view the infinite-dimensionality of functional data as a double-edged sword—on one hand, they note that the high-dimensional data samples pose challenges when developing theory, methodology and computational techniques. On the other hand, their rich structure means they naturally encode an abundance of information and can be used to answer pertinent scientific questions in diverse disciplines. Human movement biomechanics is one such discipline, where FDA can answer questions about the dynamic characteristics of a movement (e.g., "At which point in the gait cycle is the hip angle most variable?"), and how these characteristics relate to other information in the data (e.g., "Does an osteoarthritic patient's knee angle evolve differently during a gait cycle to that of a healthy control?").

1.3 Early Applications

There is a long-standing link between FDA and studies of human movement. Early methodological developments in FDA [2, 3] were motivated by the need to understand the gait of a "normal" child to make comparisons with children with walking difficulties. This was achieved using a set of biomechanical data on children's gait collected at the Motion Analysis Laboratory in the Children's Hospital, San Diego, California [6]. The data contained sagittal plane angles of the hip and knee of 39 healthy 5-year-old boys (Fig. 1.2).

Rice and Silverman [2] discussed estimation of the mean hip angle function through a spline smoothing approach [25] and proposed a leave-one-curve-out procedure (i.e., cross-validation) for selecting an appropriate level of smoothness. For estimating the covariance structure of the hip angle data, they formally extended principal component analysis (PCA) [26] to the functional setting, in what is now known as functional principal component analysis (FPCA), and demonstrated how smoothing could be incorporated into this technique. The authors also extended this method to bivariate functions, to describe how the hip and knee move simultaneously (i.e., coordinate). Leurgans et al. [3] extended canonical correlation analysis to a functional setting to demonstrate how variability in the knee angle is related to that in the hip angle. They also outlined why it is necessary to incorporate smoothing in the procedure. The work of both Rice and Silverman [2] and Leurgans et al. [3] represented significant, early methodological advancements in the field of

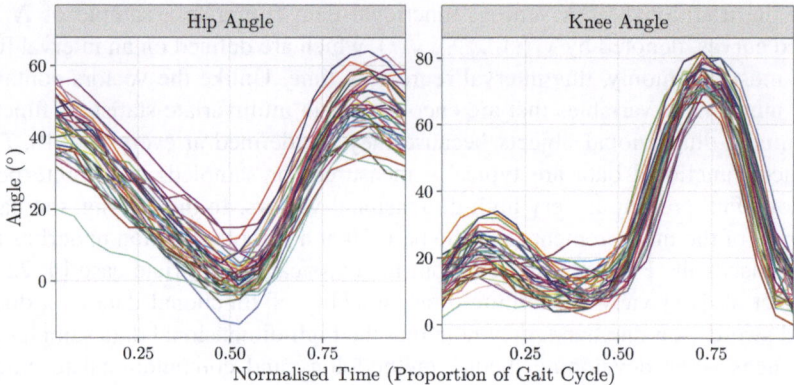

Fig. 1.2 The hip and knee angles of 39 boys from the children's gait data [2–4, 6]. **Note**: These data are publicly available in the **fda** R package

FDA and highlighted its compatibility with biomechanics and human movement as areas of application.

1.4 Recent Developments

Since these advances, FDA has been used to analyse human movement data obtained from motion analysis systems [27], force and pressure platforms [28], electromyography (EMG) [29] and sensors [15]. In a review which identified 84 FDA application articles published between 1995 and 2010, Ullah and Finch [30] found that biomechanics was the second most prevalent field of application, accounting for 11 (13%) papers included in the review. Along with applications to chewing, handwriting and pinching data, many of the biomechanics articles used FDA to study kinematics and kinetics of the lower extremities during movements such as walking and jumping. In recent years, the use of FDA for these applications has increased further. A systematic review by Dannenmaier et al. [31] comprised 13 articles where FDA was applied to walking, running or jumping movements. Other notable recent applications of FDA in human movement biomechanics include rowing [32], predicting fatigue in recreational athletes [28] and testing changes in children's gait with ankle-foot orthoses [33].

A common theme that motivates all biomechanical studies employing FDA is its ability to describe whole movements, making use of an entire time series of data by treating it as a single, smooth function. This contrasts with the traditional approach of reducing the time series down to a single scalar value for analysis, e.g., the peak knee flexion angle, before applying parametric statistical techniques (Fig. 1.3). Despite being regularly implemented in biomechanics, this approach cannot capture all of the variability within a time series and only gives a snapshot of the movement

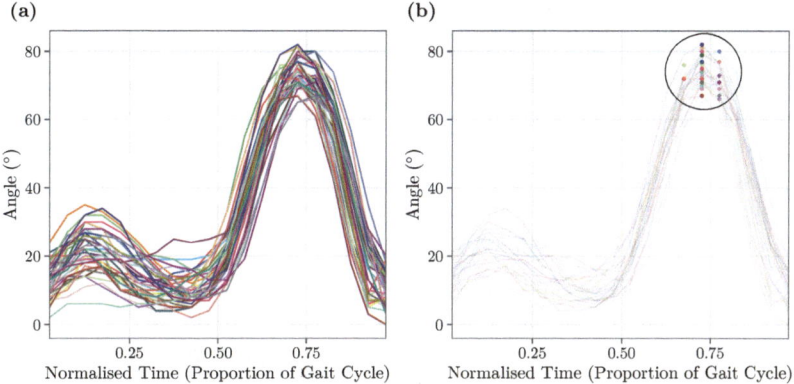

Fig. 1.3 (**a**): Functional data of the sagittal knee angle from the children's gait dataset. (**b**): The same functional data reduced to a single discrete variable—the maximum knee flexion angle. The comparison highlights the data reduction involved in converting functional data to discrete variables

at a single point in time [16]. In this regard, FDA is a state-of-the-art framework for analysing movement data, as it does not discard potentially important variability and allows for comprehensive analyses.

In addition to improving on traditional approaches, FDA also provides benefits over modern machine learning techniques. By preserving and leveraging the time-dependence in the data, FDA models estimate functional parameters that can be visualised, interpreted and understood on the same scale as the data. For example, FDA can be used to estimate a function that shows how a scalar variable (e.g., walking speed) affects knee kinematics over the course of a full gait cycle, or a function indicating which part of the gait cycle is most predictive of a certain outcome. In contrast, machine learning models that use opaque transformations of the data may have limited utility, as described by Halilaj et al. [14, p. 7]:

> If a 'black box' model predicts with high confidence that a patient will develop osteoarthritis based on their gait pattern, but offers no insight into the specific features of gait that are driving osteoarthritis progression, it is unclear how this knowledge could be used to improve the patient's health.

FDA is located at a "sweet spot" between traditional and modern modelling approaches—it can handle the high-dimensionality of continuous biomechanical data while producing transparent, interpretable models.

Despite this undoubted suitability, applications in biomechanics and human movement have not managed to stay abreast of methodological developments in FDA. That is, only elementary FDA techniques are routinely applied within the field, and the full scope of FDA is not being utilised. For example, work on multilevel [34, 35], multivariate [36–38] and phase-varying [39, 40] functional data have not made the impact in biomechanics and human movement research that they could have. Possible explanations for this are:

1. There is still a need for an accessible introduction to the full suite of FDA tools aimed at applied researchers in biomechanics and human movement research,
2. A guide for these researchers on how to use software to implement FDA methods is lacking,[1] and
3. Connections between different FDA techniques, and between these techniques and familiar statistical methods, are not well understood.

Previous review papers on FDA in biomechanics have either been systematic reviews [31] or short, tutorial-style papers focusing on specific FDA techniques [45, 46]. There are extensive monographs on FDA [e.g., 4, 20, 47], detailed review articles on FDA methodology [e.g., 21, 22, 48–51] and FDA applications in general or other fields [30, 52–54]. However, these are not pitched directly at the level of an applied researcher in biomechanics and human movement research or placed in the context of the applied field.

In this SpringerBriefs text, we provide a concise review of the functional data analysis techniques that can be used to learn from biomechanical data. We provide short, didactic introductions to several FDA techniques accompanied by real examples from biomechanics, and describe notable applications of each technique in the literature. Additionally, we discuss how these applications can be extended in light of methodological developments in FDA and emerging data in biomechanics. We do not introduce new FDA methods, nor do we aim to provide comprehensive theoretical or methodological treatments comparable to, e.g., the monograph by Ramsay and Silverman [4], though we do point the reader to where further details can be found when necessary. We provide supplementary code to reproduce every example in the review, using real and simulated data including the original children's gait dataset [2–4, 6], and the new large-scale GaitRec data [5]. Although this text is approached from an applied perspective, the inter-disciplinary examples we discuss lie at the intersection of statistics and human movement biomechanics, and we anticipate that this review will generally be of interest to researchers and practitioners in both disciplines.

---

[1] Two resources that help in this regard were published during the time spent revising this text for publication. Crainiceanu et al. [41] provide a full textbook on FDA methodology and its implementation using the **refund** [42] and **mgcv** [43] R packages (on non-biomechanics examples) with an extensive website containing computer code: https://functionaldataanalysis.org/. Gertheiss et al. [44] provide a general review of state-of-the-art FDA approaches and demonstrate them on human movement biomechanics datasets, also providing R code to replicate their examples (https://github.com/davidruegamer/FDA_tutorial). Combined with this SpringerBriefs review and associated code repository, we believe that applied researchers in biomechanics and human movement research are now better equipped with FDA tools and resources.

Bibliographic Notes

The literature review on FDA in biomechanics in Sects. 1.3–1.4 first appeared on pp. 2–4 of Edward Gunning's Ph.D. thesis [55].

Bibliographic Notes

Chapter 2
Preparing Biomechanical Data for Functional Data Analysis

Abstract This chapter describes how to transform observed biomechanical data into smooth functions using B-spline or Fourier basis function expansions, using least-squares or penalised least-squares estimation approaches. It also discusses the characteristics of certain types of biomechanical data that might make other (e.g., wavelet or FPCA) basis function approaches more suitable. The second half of this chapter introduces phase variation in biomechanical data and describes approaches for separating phase and amplitude variation via registration. Various applications of registration to biomechanical data are discussed and their findings are detailed to develop guidance on its use. Some advanced analyses of phase variation and registration techniques from the statistics literature are reviewed to highlight possibilities for future applications.

Keywords Smoothing · Basis functions · Registration · Time warping · Normalisation

2.1 Representing Biomechanical Data as Functions

In biomechanical applications, a single movement is typically one observation in the data, for example, a step or cycle starting and ending at the contact of the foot with the ground in walking or running [56, 57], a full stroke in rowing [58], or a full-hop from landing until after touch down for the one-legged hop [16]. For repeated cyclical movements such as gait, data are typically manually segmented into individual cycles based on salient features (e.g., minima, maxima or points of contact) [45]; alternatively Kurtek et al. [59] provide a quick and efficient segmentation algorithm for periodic biosignals based on methods developed for alignment (registration).

Generally, the initial step in applying FDA to biomechanics data is to convert each sequence of measurements that has been recorded throughout the movement into a smooth function [45, 46, 60]. FDA techniques often mirror analogous multivariate techniques applied to biomechanical data at discrete time points and in some situations, when pre-processing steps coincide, can yield similar or near-

© The Author(s), under exclusive license to Springer Nature Switzerland AG 2024
E. Gunning et al., *Functional Data Analysis in Biomechanics*,
SpringerBriefs in Statistics, https://doi.org/10.1007/978-3-031-68862-1_2

identical results [17]. However, representing the discrete data as a smooth function has benefits practically (e.g., it allows sampling grids to be irregular and differ between observations), methodologically (smoothing and regularisation can be incorporated at different stages of the analysis), and philosophically, as Ramsay and Dalzell [61, p. 539] remark: "some modelling problems are more natural to think through in functional terms even though only finite numbers of observations are available". Although the immediate transformation of discrete data to functions is not strictly necessary as a first step (instead, some FDA techniques involve smoothing and functional representations later in the analysis [54]), it tends to be useful and suitable for biomechanical data, so we present it as the primary approach in this section.

2.1.1   Basis Function Expansions

Basis functions provide a link between the discretely sampled measurements that we observe and the smooth underlying functions that we wish to analyse, so they are fundamental in FDA [4, 22]. We observe measurements of each function, $x(t)$, at n sampling (or discretisation) points, t_j, $j = 1, ..., n$, and we denote these measurements by $\mathbf{y} = (y_1, ..., y_n)^\top$. We assume some random error, e_j, in the measurements, giving a "signal plus noise" model

$$y_j = x(t_j) + e_j, \tag{2.1.1}$$

where $e_j \overset{i.i.d.}{\sim} \mathcal{N}(0, \sigma^2)$ [4, p. 40].[1] In this context, $x(t)$ is the underlying biomechanical signal that we wish to analyse (e.g., joint angle or force). In general, the e_j can represent measurement error or random fluctuations around a smooth underlying function [62, p. 259]. In biomechanical applications, it is natural to consider them as measurement error (or *noise*) arising from instruments (e.g., motion-capture systems, force plates or sensors) that might otherwise be removed through standard filtering techniques. If the data have already been filtered to remove the observational error, the basis function expansions we describe can still be used to convert the data to functions, but with the goal of *interpolation* rather than *smoothing* [20, p. 12].

Ramsay and Silverman [4, p. 43] define a set (or system) of basis functions $\{\phi_k(t)\}_{k=1}^K$ as a collection of known functions (i.e., they are fixed before the data analysis, rather than estimated therein), with the following two properties:

1. These functions are linearly independent (i.e., no single function in the set can be written exactly as a weighted sum of the others), and

---

[1] This notation indicates that we make the conventional regression assumption that the errors in our model arise as independent, identically distributed (i.i.d.) draws from a Gaussian (normal) distribution, with mean zero and variance σ^2.

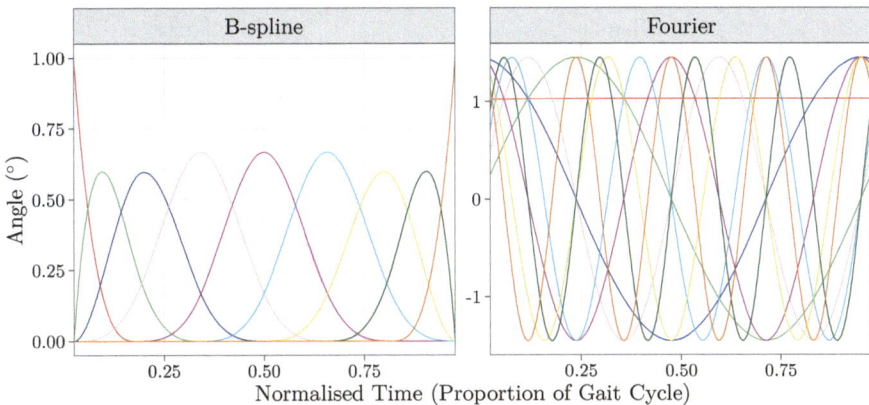

Fig. 2.1 Systems of $K = 9$ cubic B-spline (left) and Fourier (right) basis functions defined on the normalised time interval $[0, 1]$

2. A weighted sum of these functions can be used to approximate any smooth function to a desired level of accuracy, provided that the number of functions in the set (i.e., K) is made large enough.

Then, a *basis function expansion* involves expanding the function $x(t)$, in terms of a linear combination of K basis functions

$$x(t) = \sum_{k=1}^{K} c_k \phi_k(t),$$ (2.1.2)

where the vector of basis coefficients $\mathbf{c} = (c_1, \ldots, c_K)^\top$ is estimated from the data.

Biomechanical data are typically measured on a dense and equally-spaced time grid, so they can be categorised as *dense functional data* [62, 63]. Therefore, analyses of kinematic and kinetic data have primarily used B-spline or Fourier basis expansions, which are generally accepted as suitable systems of basis functions for representing smooth functions observed on moderately-dense grids [22] (Fig. 2.1). The Fourier basis is periodic—the basis functions repeat at the interval over which the basis is defined. It consists of a constant term and a sequence of trigonometric (sine and cosine) functions of increasing frequency. The periodicity of the Fourier basis has led to its use with cyclical human movements, such as gait [56, 64, 65]. The B-spline basis, a non-periodic basis system, is the most popular choice of basis for representing biomechanical data. The B-spline system is a basis of spline functions, which are piecewise polynomial functions of a specified degree, defined over sub-intervals of the domain divided by breakpoints called knots. As described by Ramsay and Silverman [4, p. 47], the adjacent polynomial segments and their derivatives up to the order one less than the polynomial degree link up smoothly at the breakpoints. For example, a cubic (degree 3) spline function's first derivative is continuous and piecewise quadratic, and its second derivative is continuous and

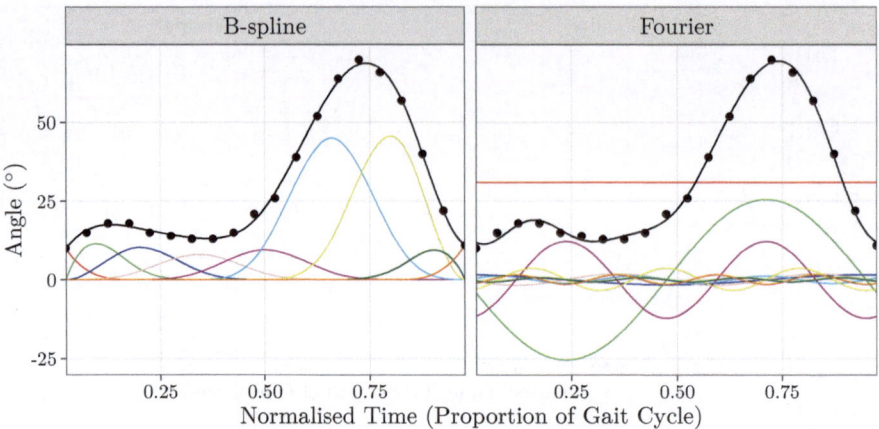

Fig. 2.2 Representation of a single knee angle curve from the children's gait dataset using the systems of cubic B-spline (left) and Fourier (right) basis functions shown in Fig. 2.1. The black points are the observed values, the black line is the fitted function and the coloured lines are the weighted basis functions

piecewise linear. The B-spline basis is constructed in such a way that each spline basis function is non-zero on a small number of intervals; this property is called *local support* [4, p. 50]. We do not provide the technical definition of the B-spline basis system here, it can be found in Eilers and Marx [66, Sect. 2] or Ramsay and Silverman [4, Sect. 3.2.5]. In biomechanical applications, B-spline basis functions have been used to represent joint angles in studies of running [16, 67, 68] and ground reaction forces [69] in jumping. Figure 2.2 shows a single curve from the children's gait dataset, modelled by B-spline and Fourier basis functions. The local support of the B-splines can be seen by two local, adjacent basis functions (blue and yellow) combining to represent the peak knee angle. The periodicity of the Fourier basis means that the start and endpoints of the fitted function match exactly at about 12.5°.

We denote the coefficients estimated from the data by $\widehat{c}_k$ and the estimate of the fitted function by $\widehat{x}(t)$. The reason for controlling the smoothness of $\widehat{x}(t)$ is conceptually clear. When observing noisy realisations of $x(t)$ as in Eq. (2.1.1), a "wiggly" (or rough) estimator $\widehat{x}(t)$ that closely follows the data will capture random variation that should be ignored. On the other hand, an estimator that is too smooth will not recover the shape of the true underlying function. The ideal scenario is somewhere in between—an estimate flexible enough to capture the true underlying function's shape without fitting to the random variation in the measurements. In statistical terms, these two competing interests are expressed in terms of the mean squared error (MSE), which is a measure of the error of $\widehat{x}(t)$ with respect to the true function $x(t)$. The MSE admits a decomposition into two separate quantities that reflect the two competing interests—the variance and the squared bias, known as the *bias-variance trade-off* [4, 70, 71]. Generally, we aim to choose a level of smoothness that should minimise the (unknown) MSE, so that our fitted function strikes the correct balance between fit to the data and smoothness.

In practice, we control the level of smoothness in two main ways. The first is to use the ordinary least squares (OLS) criterion, choosing the coefficients $\widehat{c}_k$ to minimise the sum of squared errors (SSE) from the observed data

$$\text{SSE}(\mathbf{c}) = \sum_{j=1}^{n} \left(y_j - \sum_{k=1}^{K} c_k \phi_k(t_j) \right)^2. \tag{2.1.3}$$

Smoothness is then controlled by the number of basis functions used, K. Increasing K will provide more flexibility and a wigglier fit. While some algorithms could be used to choose an optimal value for K, these can be problematic [4, p. 69]. A reasonable approach is to use different values of K and pick out the best fit by eye. An example of this in the biomechanics literature is Page et al. [72]. They carefully chose K to achieve what they considered an appropriate level of smoothing of their vertical ground reaction force data. Their work shows the fit with different values of K and justifies their choice of K.

An alternative approach, which alleviates the choosing of K and provides finer control over the level of smoothness, is to use a rich basis (large value of K) and add a penalty term to the least-squares criterion that penalises the roughness of the fitted function. With $x(t)$ as in Eq. (2.1.2), the criterion to minimise becomes

$$\text{PENSSE}_\lambda(\mathbf{c}) = \underbrace{\sum_{j=1}^{n} \left(y_j - x(t_j) \right)^2}_{\text{Fit to Data (SSE)}} + \lambda \underbrace{\text{PEN}\left(x(t) \right)}_{\substack{\text{Roughness} \\ \text{Penalty}}}. \tag{2.1.4}$$

The penalty is a regularisation term because it exploits the expected regularity (i.e., smoothness) of the function to improve estimation [4, 22]. The standard penalty is the integrated, squared second derivative of $x(t)$ as a measure of the curvature of the fitted function,[2] but other penalties can be used (e.g., if smooth derivatives are required). The smoothing parameter, λ, controls the trade-off between smoothness and fit to the data. When λ is large, more emphasis is put on minimising the penalty term and therefore controlling smoothness, whereas when λ is small, more emphasis is put on fit to the data (Fig. 2.3). We are concerned with finding the value of λ that gives optimum smoothing.

The smoothing parameter can be chosen by *cross-validation* (CV), where the data are split into two samples, training and test samples. The model is fitted to the training sample and its fit is assessed on the test sample. This is repeated for different training and test samples called *folds* and performed for a range of values

---

[2] This is considered a measure of curvature because a straight line is perfectly smooth and its second derivative is exactly zero [4, p. 84].

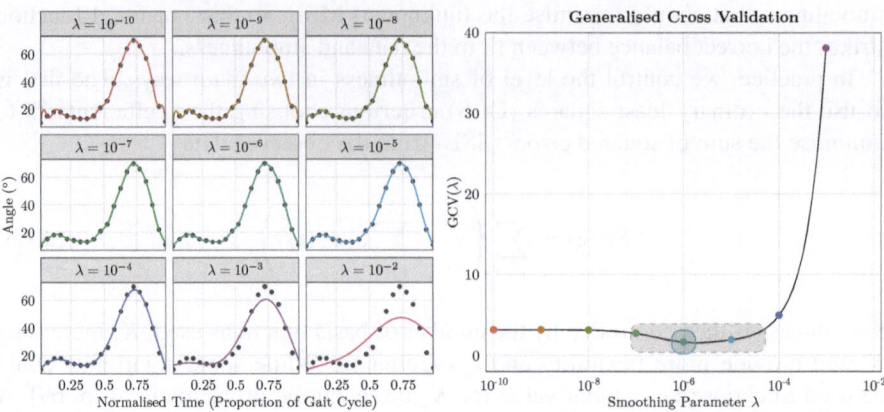

Fig. 2.3 **Left**: Smoothing of a single knee angle curve from the children's gait dataset using $K = 20$ B-spline basis functions and values of λ varying on a $\log_{10}$ scale. **Right**: Demonstration of a grid search using GCV to determine the optimal value of λ, where the optimal value at $\lambda = 10^{-6}$ is highlighted in turquoise. A region of potential values for λ around the optimal value, about which a more refined grid search could be conducted or a subjective choice could be made, is shaded in grey

of λ. The value of λ that gives the lowest error on the test set, averaged over all folds, is chosen. A more popular alternative, which does not require splitting the data and re-smoothing many times, is *generalised cross-validation* (GCV) [73] (Fig. 2.3). It is a measure of fit to the data, that is "discounted" to account for the wiggliness (or "complexity") of the fitted curve [4, p. 97]. The value of λ that minimises the GCV criterion is chosen (Fig. 2.3). In addition to the reduced computational overhead, it is less likely than CV to under-smooth the data [4, 74]. A final alternative to CV and GCV is a maximum likelihood approach. This involves viewing the penalised criterion in Eq. (2.1.4) as the log-likelihood of a linear mixed effects model [75, 76], so that the smoothing parameter and basis coefficients can be estimated "automatically" simply by fitting that model, typically by restricted maximum likelihood (REML) (see [43, 71, 77, 78]). Coffey [79] demonstrated this approach for modelling biomechanical joint angle data in running—it is especially useful because it avoids trialling different values of λ manually.

Of course, there is no universally best choice of basis expansion or smoothing approach. However, B-spline basis functions and smoothing with a roughness penalty offer a reasonably flexible and efficient way to represent the data encountered in many biomechanical applications. B-splines are not tied to the periodicity of the data and with enough basis functions, they can represent local functional behaviour well. The roughness penalty approach allows fine control over the level of smoothness—there are several ways of choosing the smoothing parameter and it can also be adjusted by eye to give the desired level of smoothness[3] (Fig. 2.3). The order of the B-spline basis and the order of the roughness penalty can also be easily tailored to facilitate smooth estimates of the first and second derivatives of the fitted functions. In biomechanical applications, this allows for suitable functional estimates of velocity and acceleration from observed displacement data, which are often useful quantities in describing a movement.

An exception is electromyography (EMG) data, which have temporally localised features, appearing as sharp, high-frequency "spikes", that are difficult to model with B-spline or Fourier bases in the absence of other pre-processing. To deal with these features, Allison et al. [80] used a wavelet representation of EMG data to compare muscle activity patterns between individuals with gluteal tendinopathy and healthy controls. There has been limited use of wavelet basis functions in applications to biomechanics to date, but they provide an interesting avenue to explore for researchers who wish to model EMG data. Wavelet basis functions are jointly indexed by time and frequency and are used to decompose complex signals. They have been used successfully as the basis functions for functional data analyses in other biomedical fields [22, 81] and Morris [22, p. 327] notes that they are well suited to functions with "spikes, discontinuities and other non-stationary features". In addition, there are fast algorithms for computing the wavelet basis coefficients, which may provide an advantage over the least-squares approaches when the grid of time points on which the data are observed is very large (i.e., if the biomechanical data are sampled at a very high frequency). We do not give an example wavelet representation of biomechanical data, but we point the reader to work by Pigoli and Sangalli [82] on modelling electrocardiogram (ECG) measurements, which possess similar characteristics to EMG data.

The dense sampling scheme (or *resolution*) of biomechanical data contrasts with sparse and irregularly sampled functional data, where each curve can only be realised at a limited number of points. This commonly occurs in longitudinal studies, where a small number of measurements are available at irregular intervals (e.g., bone mineral density measured for a group of females at different ages in James and Sugar [83]). With few observations per curve, expansions onto a rich, pre-specified basis (e.g., Fourier or B-spline), as we have described, may not be possible, so this type of data motivated the Principal Analysis by Conditional Estimation (PACE) algorithm [84]. In PACE, a functional principal components (FPCs) basis is estimated from the data—a small number of these basis functions can capture most of the variation in the curves—and FPC score estimates are obtained by a conditioning step, allowing smooth representations of functional data with small numbers of irregular measurements per-subject [84]. As Halilaj et al. [14, p. 7] note, the ability to impute missing parts of partially-observed curves is likely to become even more important for human movement biomechanists in the future, due to the

---

[3] Adjusting the smoothing parameter by eye allows the biomechanist to use domain-specific knowledge on the smoothness of the underlying process, making sure key features of a movement are not under-smoothed or smoothed out.

proliferation of data from wearable sensors which often contain missing fragments (presenting as "gaps") due to device non-wear.

2.2 Registration

2.2.1 Phase Variation in Biomechanical Data

Samples of functional data typically exhibit variation in amplitude (such as peak heights), called *amplitude variation*, and in the horizontal direction (such as peak timings), referred to as *phase* (or *horizontal* or *timing*) *variation* [62]. Most statistical analyses of curve data rely on the calculation of cross-sectional (or "point-by-point") means, either explicitly or implicitly, and the presence of phase variation can mean a loss of interpretation and statistical efficiency [7, p. 1698]. When key characteristics such as the positions of peaks are misaligned between curves, these characteristics will be dampened or distorted (and therefore no longer interpretable or representative) when the mean is calculated at each grid point [62]; a simulated example is shown in Fig. 2.4. Statistical analyses will also be inefficient due to the variability introduced by the temporal misalignments. A mean that truly reflects the shape and features of a group of curves is called a *structural mean*. This phenomenon is well understood in biomechanics. For example, Dos'Santos et al. [85] demonstrated that discrete points taken from an averaged movement profile can be significantly smaller in magnitude than the average of the same discrete points across all trials.

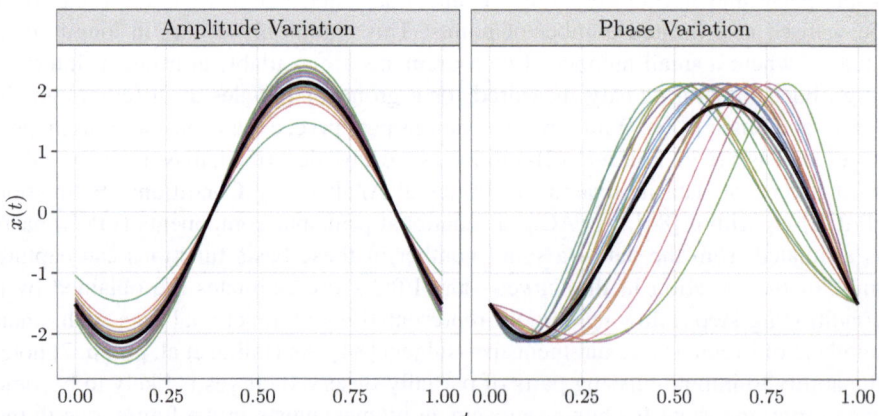

Fig. 2.4 Simulated functional data exhibiting only amplitude variation (left) and phase variation (right). The coloured lines are individual functions in the sample and the thick black line is the cross-sectional mean. For the functions with phase variation, the mean is not representative of any one function. **Note**: The data were simulated using the **registr** R package [86]

2.2.2 Description of Registration

Registration (also known as *alignment, warping* or *synchronisation*) is concerned with the identification and separation of amplitude and phase variability in functional data. Given a sample of N functional data $x_1(t), ..., x_N(t)$ defined on the interval $[0, T]$, Kneip and Ramsay [87] formulate the registration problem as the search for a set of smooth, strictly monotonic functions h_i such that functions of the form

$$x^*(t) = x\big(h(t)\big) = x \circ h(t) \qquad (2.2.1)$$

have their features aligned. The *warping function* $h(t)$ represents timing variation. In biomechanical applications, it can be thought of as a mapping between physical time and, as Ramsay and Silverman [4, p. 128] describe, some biological time scale "that can be non-linearly related to physical time and can vary from case to case". Therefore, we require $h(t)$ to be monotonically increasing, that is, for $s, t \in [0, T]$ if $s < t$ then $h(s) < h(t)$, since it does not make sense for time to go backwards on either scale [20, p. 120]. Most registration procedures, aside from scattered exceptions such as the work of Sangalli et al. [39], register functions to a common interval such that $h(0) = 0$ and $h(T) = T$ [20, p. 120]. For functions observed on different intervals, $[0, T_i]$, this is $h_i(0) = 0$ and $h_i(T) = T_i$ for all i. To visualise a warping function, time can be subtracted, giving $h(t) - t$. This is called a *deformation function* and represents the perturbation to time by the warping function. We call $x^*(t)$ a "registered" function.

Landmark registration was one of the earliest registration techniques developed [88, 89] and it is still used today [90]. In landmark registration, special features, such as peak locations or zero crossings in the functions or their derivatives, called landmarks, are aligned to a target location [62].[4] A common target is the average landmark time [20, 62]. The warping functions are smooth, strictly increasing, non-linear transformations that map the target to the landmark timings. Wang et al. [62, p. 283] state that landmark registration is a "gold standard" registration method in settings where common landmarks are clearly identifiable in each curve. We illustrate landmark registration in Fig. 2.5. We have chosen a single landmark per curve, the peak knee flexion angle, identified as the zero-crossing of the first derivative with a negative slope in the second half of the gait cycle. However, multiple landmarks per curve can be used if they are identifiable.

Landmark registration is not suitable if landmarks are not identifiable in all curves. For example, they might be missing, or hard to identify in some functions [62], or features might differ between groups in the data. In addition, landmarks often have to be identified manually, which is laborious if the number of curves is large. These reasons have motivated the development of more refined techniques,

---

[4] Definition adapted from Wang et al. [21].

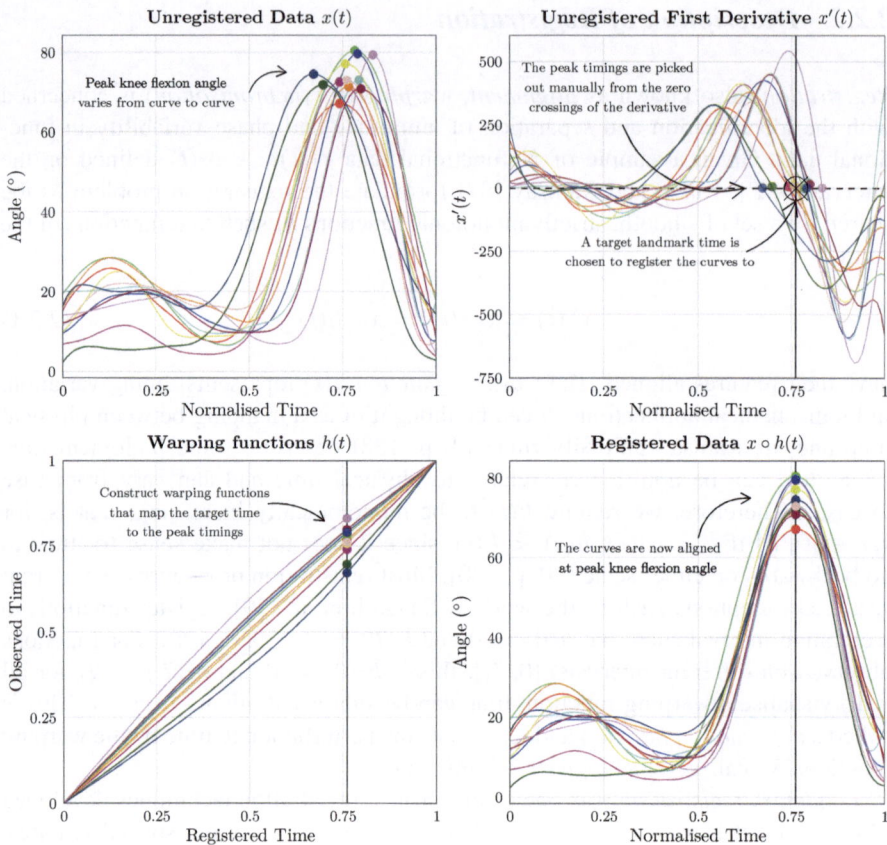

Fig. 2.5 A graphical representation of landmark registration on gait data exhibiting (simulated) phase variation

called continuous registration methods, that align entire curves rather than specified points [20]. Continuous registration is an active area of research, where most approaches find warping functions that maximise (or minimise) measures of similarity (or dissimilarity) between registered functions. It is important to note that simply minimising the squared distance

$$\|x_0 - x \circ h\|^2 = \int_0^T \Big(x_0(t) - x\big(h(t)\big)\Big)^2 \mathrm{d}t \qquad (2.2.2)$$

to register a function $x(t)$ to a target function $x_0(t)$ will give undesirable warping (known as pinching) if flexible warping functions are allowed [4, p. 138][91]. Therefore, continuous registration techniques consider both the similarity measure being optimised and the family of warping functions used. Examples of continuous registration techniques include Ramsay and Silverman [4], Sangalli et al. [39], Kneip and Ramsay [87], Srivastava et al. [92], Wagner and Kneip [93].

2.2.3 Applications of Registration in Biomechanics Research

Most FDA techniques require all functions in the data to be defined on the same interval (known as the domain) [45]. In biomechanics, the time taken to complete a movement can vary from individual to individual and from trial to trial. Therefore, it is commonplace to perform *linear time* (or *length*) *normalisation* as a first step, to linearly stretch or compress each domain so that the start and end points are aligned. This is a basic form of registration because it aligns the curves through a transformation of time. Honert and Pataky [94] demonstrated that the choice of the start and end points of a gait cycle used in normalisation can impact the outcomes of an analysis.

Beyond linear time normalisation, registration is not always used in applications of FDA to biomechanics. A possible explanation is that, although a certain level of phase variation is often present in biomechanical data after time normalisation, standard tools (e.g., functional principal components analysis) typically still work reasonably well in the absence of registration, and it may be deemed unnecessarily complex. The reduction in variability achieved through successful registration should, however, incentivise its use. For example, it has been noted that registered curves usually require fewer functional principal components to describe them and these are usually easier to interpret [91, 95]. Landmark registration has typically been preferred to continuous registration, possibly due to the tractability of the approach and the availability of biomechanically meaningful landmarks to register to. Landmark registration has been applied in biomechanics and human movement research to align data from the one-legged hop at maximum knee flexion angle during take-off and landing phase, and at touch down [16], the drop-jump at touch down, take-off and minimal pelvis position [67], gait at initial contact and toe-off [96] and bilateral and unilateral jumps at the end of the deceleration phase [69].

Registration is sensitive to the characteristics of the data. As Crane et al. [97] note, the successful application of registration to biomechanical data typically depends on the prominence of well-defined features (e.g., peaks, troughs, valleys and zero-crossings) in the set of curves, which, in general, will vary with the movement and data type. Therefore, studies have assessed the utility of registration in specific biomechanical applications. Generally, they have been in favour of registration or have acknowledged its utility. We discuss some of the assessments below.

By landmark registering muscle power curves of twenty healthy subjects during gait, Sadeghi et al. [98] found increased peak mean powers and reduced inter-subject variability, without any noticeable distortions of curves shapes. They therefore recommended the application of registration when analysing movement data on able-bodied gait. Page et al. [72] showed the utility of registration for vertical ground reaction force data during the sit-to-stand movement. Using the continuous registration method of Ramsay and Silverman [4] in a two-step approach, they found that inter- and intra-individual variability was reduced with no apparent changes in the shapes of the functions. Ryan et al. [27] studied knee kinematics in the vertical jump and found that landmark registration allowed for more interpretable features to be extracted with functional principal components analysis. Crane et al. [97] used the continuous registration method of Ramsay and Silverman [4] to register cyclical chewing data from 22 subjects. They observed little difference in mean curves before and after registration and found that warping functions were linear, indicating registration added little to linear time normalisation. However, they acknowledged that the reduction in variability could justify registration prior to applying other FDA techniques. Moudy et al. [99] and White et al. [100] found that landmark registration of vertical ground reaction force data improved predictive performance of measures of countermovement jump performance. Zin et al. [90] investigated the use of landmark registration and the continuous registration method of Ramsay and Silverman [4], separately and in combination on kinematic data of recreational athletes performing the American kettlebell swing. All three approaches that they used (landmark, continuous and landmark then continuous) increased peaks in mean curves, reduced inter-subject and intra-subject variability, and improved statistical power to detect between-group differences. Combining the techniques, performing landmark followed by continuous registration, worked best.

Conventional techniques used to remove phase variation in biomechanical data are also forms of registration (see Helwig et al. [101] for a short, practical communication of these techniques). For example, dynamic time warping (DTW) is a discrete registration, used to find warping functions that pass linearly through the discretisation points and minimise the squared distance between registered sequences of points [91, 102]. Another example, piecewise linear length normalisation (PLLN) [101], is a special case of landmark registration with piecewise linear warping functions. Piecewise linearity might be sufficient to remove phase variability, but it might also be important to represent the warping functions using techniques from FDA to impose desirable properties. For example, basis function representations can be constructed to enforce smoothness and monotonicity for interpretable warping functions that can be used in further analysis, and differentiability so that the derivatives of registered functions can be analysed (see Marron et al. [91], Sect. 3.5). This reflects the more general reason for considering registration within the FDA paradigm—phase variation is treated as *functional*, and it is defined and modelled in the warping functions rather than being removed as a pre-processing step. Human movement biomechanics is an area in which understanding both amplitude and timing variation is crucial [7, 72], and one where "phase variation should be viewed and studied as a substantively interesting part of the total picture, rather than as an ignorable nuisance" [103, p. 1874]. Registration with FDA makes a joint analysis of amplitude and phase possible.

With this in mind, we finish this section with a synopsis of papers from The Electronic Journal of Statistics' special issue on Statistics of Time Warpings and Phase Variations (Volume 8, Number 2, 2014), which provides a rich resource on

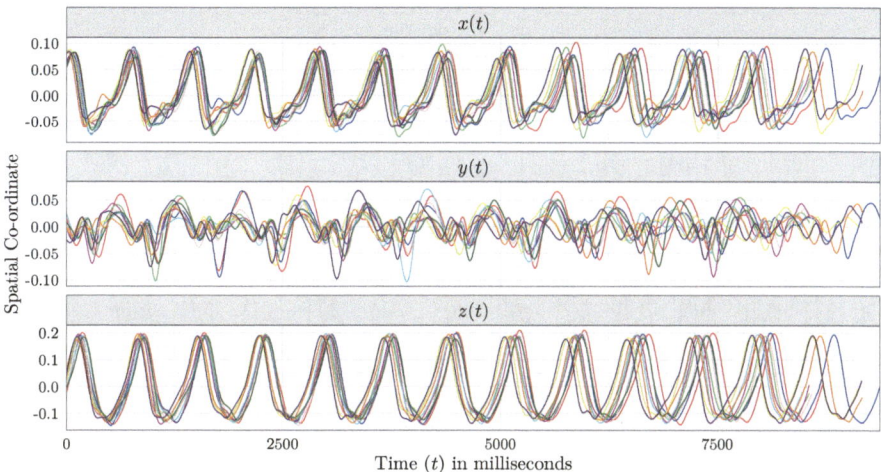

Fig. 2.6 The three-dimensional coordinates of the juggling data before any registration was performed. Each coloured line is a different trial. **Note**: The juggling dataset is available at https://github.com/FAST-ULxNUIG/SpringerBriefs/tree/main/chapter-02/juggling-data

phase variation in FDA. This special issue disseminates results of a workshop held at the Mathematical Biosciences Institute in Ohio State University [104] that analysed four functional datasets exhibiting phase variation. Marron et al. [7] describe the workshop and a review of the registration literature. We restrict our commentary to the biomechanical data analysed in the workshop, the juggling data. The dataset contains the x, y, z coordinates of a juggler's index finger as they juggled three balls, captured using infra-red emitting diodes [7]. It consists of 10 juggling trials, each lasting 10 seconds, with between 10 and 13 full cycles per trial (Fig. 2.6). Ramsay et al. [8] describe the data collection and processing, and provide some initial perspectives on the data. The analyses of phase variation investigated the ways in which tempo, rhythm and control vary in juggling.

Ramsay et al. [105] applied landmark registration and continuous registration [4] to one-dimensional tangential velocities of the full trials. They landmark registered peaks representing the ball leaving the hand ("launch peak velocities") to equidistant points (Fig. 2.7). Subsequent continuous registration towards a periodic function revealed a biphasic timing pattern within cycles, reflecting the ball's trajectory and the brain's ability to react. Bernardi et al. [106] used the functional k-means alignment algorithm [39] to simultaneously register and cluster the three-dimensional coordinates of individual juggling cycles. In this method, the warping functions are shifts and stretches of the domain, the algorithm does not require functions to share a common domain (pre or post-registration), and simultaneously clustering and registering to different templates ensures groups of curves with different features are not forced to be aligned. Poss and Wagner [95] also combined modelling and registration, using the method of Kneip and Ramsay [87] to register the three-dimensional coordinates to (multivariate) functional principal components

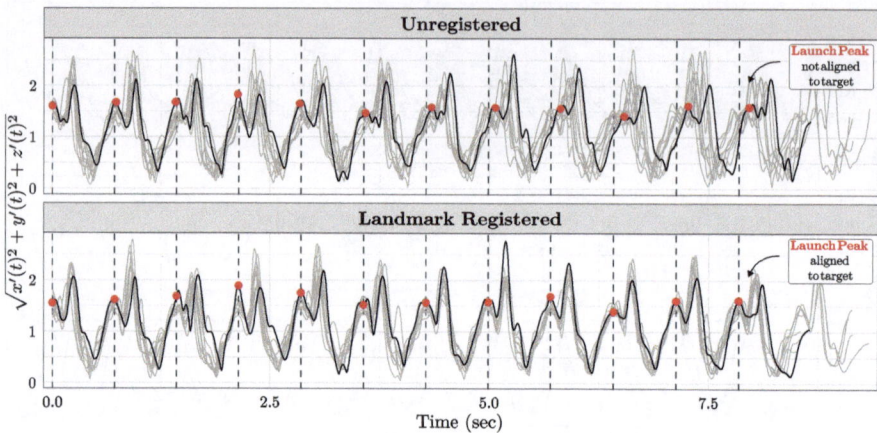

Fig. 2.7 The grey lines show the tangential velocities of the unregistered (top) and landmark registered (bottom) juggling data. The first trial is highlighted in black and its launch peaks are shown as red dots. The launch peaks were aligned to equally spaced points (dashed grey vertical lines) for each trial. **Note**: This landmark registration analysis of Ramsay et al. [105] was replicated manually using the juggling data and some code provided by Prof. Ramsay. As such, it may not be identical to the results presented by these authors but serves to demonstrate their main ideas

(FPCs), which represented common features to be aligned. Lu and Marron [107] and Kurtek et al. [108] used the elastic functional data analysis framework [92] to align the juggling data. This framework aligns functions based their square-root velocity function (SRVF) representation and has been shown to compare favourably with existing registration techniques on real and simulated datasets (see Srivastava et al. [40]). Lu and Marron [107] used this method to register and cluster the one-dimensional tangential acceleration functions, and Kurtek et al. [108] registered the three-dimensional coordinates of the juggling data to produce generative models for visualising amplitude and phase variation. Finally, Brunel and Park [109] used a technique from shape analysis, called the "Frenet-Serret representation" [110], to define a structural mean for the three-dimensional coordinates *without* performing registration.

This brief synopsis highlights the wide array of tools that have been developed to deal with phase variation in biomechanical data. The approaches varied not only in their registration techniques, but also in the unit (e.g., full trials or individual cycles) and the goals (e.g., description of phase variation, clustering of cycles or estimation of a structural mean) of the analysis. While some of the findings overlapped— Ramsay et al. [105] and Kurtek et al. [108] found similar patterns of phase variation within a cycle and the clusters found by Bernardi et al. [106] and Lu and Marron [107] were reasonably similar—it highlights that there is no "correct" answer to problems of this type, and different approaches can uncover different patterns in the data.

2.2.4 A Final Word on the Registration of Biomechanical Data

In summary, landmark registration, and to a lesser extent continuous registration, have been shown to work well when used to reduce phase variation in biomechanical data. Moving forward, efforts should be made to incorporate the treatment of phase variation into the data analysis pipeline rather than discard it as a pre-processing step, ideally through joint models with amplitude. The applications to the juggling data show how this can be achieved and what it can reveal about timing in a movement. Admittedly, some of these techniques are advanced, and therefore we have provided a short description of their application to highlight them as possibilities, rather than present the mathematics that underlie them (for more in-depth summaries, see Marron et al. [91], Ramsay [103]). It also must be acknowledged that registration of functional data is an area still very much under development and many open questions remain (see Marron et al. [91], Sect. 1.3). As Marron et al. [91] explain, there is no universal solution to the registration problem, i.e., no one method is guaranteed to perform well, or even be suitable, in all situations. This arises, in part, because phase and amplitude variation are not universally defined as concepts, and instead they exist within the context of the data being analysed and the objectives of the analysis—the differing findings from the analyses of the juggling data evidence this point. As such, we are unable to provide a general recommendation on how to treat phase variation in biomechanical data, but the literature we have reviewed should provide some guidance. A takeaway is that registration must be applied to biomechanical data with caution [27, 99], and in general, it is advisable to run subsequent data analyses with and without registration to assess the sensitivity of the results. We envisage registration of biomechanical and human movement data being most effective when subject matter experts, like clinicians, coaches or practitioners, engage in the data analysis to contextually define phase and amplitude variation. A translational challenge lies in finding practical, comprehensible ways to visualise and communicate phase variation in biomechanical data, akin to how amplitude variation is explored with functional principal components analysis.

Bibliographic Notes

- Text and examples in this chapter first appeared in Chap. 2 of Edward Gunning's Ph.D. thesis [55]. In particular, versions of Figs. 2.1, 2.2, 2.3, 2.4 and 2.5 appeared on p. 18, p. 19, p. 23, p. 26 and p. 28 of the thesis, respectively.
- The idea of representing the discrete data as smooth functions as an immediate first step is central to the FDA philosophy presented throughout Ramsay and Silverman's book [4]. As such, methodological descriptions in Sect. 2.1 summarise more extensive treatments provided in Ramsay and Silverman [4, Chaps. 3–5, pp. 37–109].

- Likewise, descriptions of registration are based on more methodological works by Ramsay and Silverman [4, Chap. 7, pp. 127–171], Ramsay et al. [20, Chap. 8, pp. 117–130] and Wang et al. [62, Sect. 5.2].
- All papers analysing the juggling data are contained in the "Special Section on Statistics of Time Warpings and Phase Variations", Volume 8, Issue Number 2 of the Electronic Journal of Statistics (2014).

Chapter 3
Exploring Variation in Biomechanical Data

Abstract Exploring variation is often the goal when researchers apply the tools of functional data analysis to biomechanical data. This chapter describes functional summary statistics, such as the mean and covariance functions, as a first step for this purpose. Then, visualisation tools for functional data analysis, which are useful for understanding variability and structure in functional data, are reviewed. Finally, this chapter discusses functional principal components analysis, a method that is frequently applied to biomechanical data to explore variation, providing an in-depth overview of its use in biomechanics research and discussing its extensions for modern biomechanical data. The methods outlined in each section of this chapter are accompanied by practical example demonstrations on the GaitRec dataset.

Keywords Functional principal components analysis · Functional boxplot · Summary statistics

3.1 Summary Statistics and Visualisation

Summary statistics and visualisation techniques can be used to summarise data structures, identify important details and characteristics and guide subsequent data analysis and modelling. These tools, which generally fall under the umbrella of *exploratory data analysis*, are especially useful for functional data because of their natural high-dimensionality and intricate structure [111, p. 116]. Summary statistics and visualisation are dynamic components of an iterative data analysis. For example, we typically use visualisation before registration to assess whether it is required and also afterwards to diagnose whether it has been successful.

3.1.1 Functional Summary Statistics

Classical univariate and multivariate summary statistics have functional analogues [4, pp. 22–26]. Given a sample of N functional data $x_1(t), ..., x_N(t)$ on the interval

© The Author(s), under exclusive license to Springer Nature Switzerland AG 2024   25
E. Gunning et al., *Functional Data Analysis in Biomechanics*,
SpringerBriefs in Statistics, https://doi.org/10.1007/978-3-031-68862-1_3

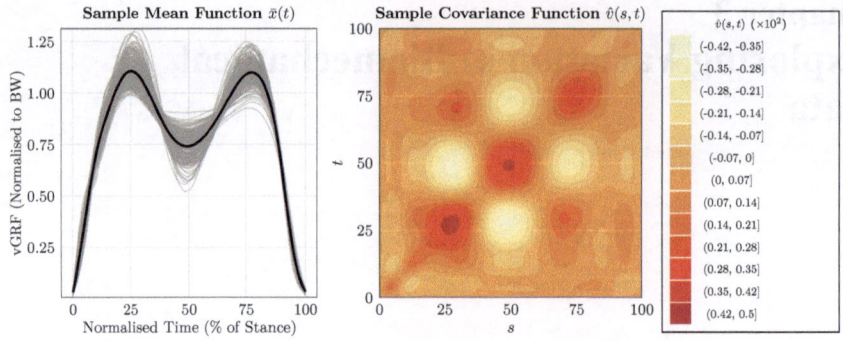

Fig. 3.1 **Left:** The sample mean vGRF function for a sample of healthy controls from the GaitRec dataset in black overlaid on the individual curves in grey. **Right:** The sample covariance function for the same sample of curves

$[0, T]$, the sample mean function

$$\bar{x}(t) = \frac{1}{N} \sum_{i=1}^{N} x_i(t) \tag{3.1.1}$$

is the sample mean average of all curves in the dataset at a given point $t \in [0, T]$ [4, p. 22]. The mean vertical ground reaction force (vGRF) for a sample of healthy controls from the GaitRec dataset is shown in the left panel of Fig. 3.1. The data have been time normalised, and a light continuous registration applied, to ensure the mean is representative of the sample. It shows peaks at about 25 and 75% of the gait cycle, with a dip in between. The mean is overlaid on the individual curves, coloured light grey, which is a useful way to assess its representativeness, and where the variation about it lies.

For multivariate data, co-variation among several variables is summarised by the covariance *matrix*. Analogously, variation in a sample of functional data is represented by the sample covariance *function*

$$\hat{v}(s, t) = \frac{1}{N - 1} \sum_{i=1}^{N} (x_i(s) - \bar{x}(s)) (x_i(t) - \bar{x}(t)), \tag{3.1.2}$$

for $s, t \in [0, T]$. The function $\hat{v}(s, t)$ summarises co-variation (or dependence) between the function values at argument values s, t. For identical argument values, $\hat{v}(t, t)$ is the sample variance

$$\widehat{\text{Var}}(t) = \frac{1}{N - 1} \sum_{i=1}^{N} (x_i(t) - \bar{x}(t))^2, \tag{3.1.3}$$

at the point t. As a function on a two-dimensional domain (i.e., a surface), we can visualise $\hat{v}(s, t)$ as a contour plot, a filled-contour plot or as a three-dimensional surface plot. The right panel of Fig. 3.1 shows a filled-contour plot of the covariance function for the sample of healthy controls from the GaitRec dataset. The x- and y-axes represent argument values s, t and the colour represents the value of $\hat{v}(s, t)$—the colour scale ranges from yellow (negative covariance) to dark red (positive covariance). Along the diagonal from the bottom left to the top right, the sample variance for identical argument values ($s = t$) can be seen. This variance is largest at 25, 50 and 75% of the gait cycle (the darkest red), which correspond to the timings of the two peaks and the valley in the middle of the cycle. Looking at the individual functions (grey lines) in the left panel of Fig. 3.1, this is indeed where most of the variation in the data lies. Interestingly, a negative covariance around $\hat{v}(25, 50)$ and $\hat{v}(50, 75)$ can be seen. This indicates an inverse relationship (or negative dependence) between the height of the peaks and the height of the valley (or "dip") in the middle. That is, higher-than-average peaks seem to be related to a lower-than-average dip. Finally, it is worth noting that $\hat{v}(s, t) = \hat{v}(t, s)$—the covariance function is *symmetric*.

The sample covariance function $\hat{v}(s, t)$ can be normalised to give the sample correlation function

$$\widehat{\text{Cor}}(s, t) = \frac{\hat{v}(s, t)}{\sqrt{\widehat{\text{Var}}(s)\widehat{\text{Var}}(t)}}, \tag{3.1.4}$$

which is the functional analogue of the sample correlation matrix in multivariate statistics. The covariance function can be extended to summarise dependence between pairs of functions (e.g., hip and knee angles, see Ramsay and Silverman [4, p. 24]), and thus used to summarise the dependence in samples of multivariate functional data (see Chap. 6).

3.1.2 Visualisation Tools for Functional Data

As is the case for summary statistics, analogues of visualisation tools for scalar (or multivariate) data can be used to explore functional data. However, the tools may not be directly or immediately translatable to the functional setting and need to be adapted [112]. For example, the *boxplot*, which was introduced by Tukey [113, pp. 39–41] over 40 years ago, is still one of the most widely-used graphical techniques today [114]. The classical boxplot provides a five-number summary for a sample of scalar data: the median, the first quartile, the third quartile, the minimum and the maximum [112] (the minimum and maximum are usually calculated from all data lying within "fences" 1.5 times the interquartile range from the hinges of the box, with values lying outside these fences flagged as potential outliers) (Fig. 3.2). However, the constitution of a median, quartile or maximum is not immediately obvious when the data are *curves*, rather than scalar values. For functional data,

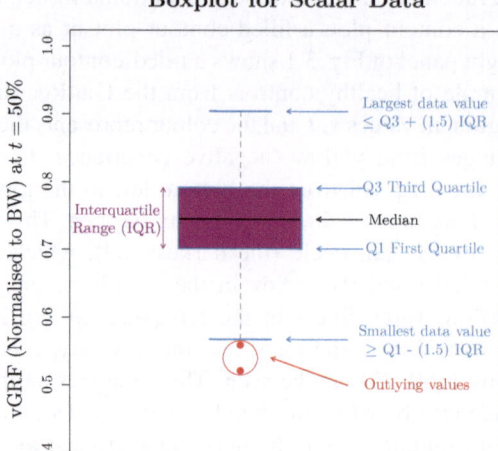

Fig. 3.2 A boxplot of scalar values from the vGRF data of healthy controls used in Fig. 3.1. The scalar data was obtained by choosing the vGRF value at 50% of the gait cycle for each curve

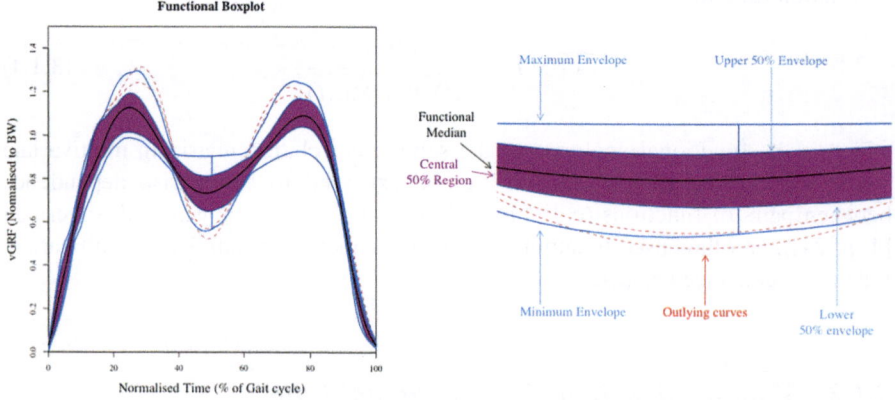

Fig. 3.3 **Left**: A functional boxplot of the vGRF data from healthy individuals. It is coloured analogously to the classical boxplot in Fig. 3.2 for interpretation. **Right**: A focused view of the functional boxplot from the left panel with the important aspects labelled. **Note**: The fbplot() function in the **fda** R package was used to construct the boxplot

there is no unique ranking of observations, so the idea of *functional data depth*, which aims to generalise the notion of ranking or ordering to a functional setting, must be used [112, 115]. We do not discuss different definitions of functional data depth here, but popular definitions can be found in [116] and [115, Sect. 2]

The functional boxplot of Sun and Genton [117] is one of the primary functional data visualisation tools, and it is implemented in the **fda** R package [118]. The left panel of Fig. 3.3 contains a functional boxplot of the vGRF data from healthy individuals, with the right panel providing a concentrated view of the central portion for closer inspection. The features in the functional boxplot are coloured to match the colours of analogous features in the classical boxplot shown in Fig. 3.2. The functional boxplot requires that a functional depth providing a center-outward ordering of the sample of curves $x_{[1]}(t), \ldots, x_{[N]}(t)$ is defined. With this ordering, $x_{[1]}(t)$ is the most "central" curve with the largest depth value and is called the *functional median* [112]. Like in the classical boxplot, it is represented by a black line in the centre of the graphic (Fig. 3.3).

Next, upper and lower 50% envelopes are constructed to define the central 50% region; the envelopes are analogous to the lower and upper quartiles which define the top and bottom box hinges in the classical boxplot, and the central 50% region is the functional analogue of the box which spans the interquartile range [117]. Mathematically, Sun and Genton [117] define this region as

$$C_{0.5} = \{(t, x(t)) : \min_{r=1,\ldots,\lfloor n/2 \rfloor} x_{[r]}(t) \leq x(t) \leq \max_{r=1,\ldots,\lfloor n/2 \rfloor} x_{[r]}(t)\}, \qquad (3.1.5)$$

where $\lfloor n/2 \rfloor$ is the smallest whole number greater than or equal to $n/2$ [112, 117].

More intuitively, Eq. (3.1.5) means that the curves are arranged in descending order based on their functional depth, and the top 50% of them are gathered—this subset represents the half of the dataset that are the "most central". From this subset, the upper and lower 50% envelopes are "traced out" as the minimum and maximum values, respectively, of all curves in this subset at each point in the time domain. Unlike the functional median, which is a single curve from the sample, the envelopes are carved out from pieces of different curves and do not correspond to any one curve [112]. The central 50% region is shown in purple in Fig. 3.3, enclosed by the upper and lower 50% envelopes in light blue. The minimum and maximum envelopes are indicated by the outer light blue lines and are traced out similarly, but from the whole sample, with potential outlying curves removed. The outlying curves are detected analogously to in the classical boxplot: the central 50% region is extended by 1.5 times its range at each point in the time domain, and curves that lie outside this fence at *any* point in the domain are identified as potential outliers [112, 117]. The minimum and maximum envelopes are shown and labelled in light blue in Fig. 3.3, with two outlying curves represented as dashed red lines.

Further descriptions of the functional boxplot and its extensions, with examples using the children's gait data, can be found in a review of functional data visualisation by Genton and Sun [112]. Hyndman and Shang [115] also review and propose alternative visualisation tools for functional data, such as *functional bagplots*, and demonstrate their ability to detect curves that lie outside the typical range of the data ("magnitude outliers") and curves that exhibit non-typical shapes ("shape outliers"). Although exploring variation in the data and identifying and understanding idiosyncrasies is often the goal when the tools of FDA are applied to biomechanical data, the functional visualisation tools developed by Sun and Genton [117], Hyndman and Shang [115] and others have not been used widely in biomechanics applications. Additionally, their associated outlier detection capabilities could be used to detect erroneous kinematic data arising from, e.g., marker misplacement, when preparing large-scale biomechanical datasets. While the aforementioned visualisation tools are accompanied by software implementations to produce static graphics, it is also worth mentioning the *interactive* visualisation tools provided by Wrobel et al. [111] in the **refund.shiny** R package [119]. This package generates an interactive environment to visualise the results of common FDA methods that can be applied using the **refund** R package [42], and is especially useful when visualisation is required for model checking and building.

3.2 Functional Principal Components Analysis

3.2.1 Description and Application to the GaitRec Data

Functional principal components analysis (FPCA) is the most widely-used FDA technique [62] and it is also the one that is most frequently applied to biomechanical data. FPCA can be introduced in a number of ways. We provide a shortened version of the description of FPCA provided in Ramsay and Silverman [4, pp. 149–151] and Ramsay et al. [20, pp. 100–102], motivated as an extension of classical multivariate PCA to the functional setting. For a more mathematical perspective, see Horváth and Kokoszka [120].

We define FPCA as the search for weight functions $\widehat{\xi}_1(t), ..., \widehat{\xi}_R(t)$, that reveal the most variation in the data, also referred to as the dominant modes of variation. These weight functions can be used to visualise and understand the covariance structure in a way that is more intuitive than the visualisation of $\hat{v}(s, t)$ that we presented in Fig. 3.1 [53][4, p. 147]. Directly analogous to classical multivariate PCA, we are interested in variation around the sample mean function $\overline{x}(t)$, so it is typically subtracted prior to FPCA [20, p. 100]. The rth (sample) functional principal component (FPC) $\widehat{\xi}_r(t)$ is defined as the weight function that maximises the variation in the FPC scores defined by

$$\widehat{f_{ir}} = \int_0^T \widehat{\xi}_r(t) \, (x_i(t) - \bar{x}(t)) \, \mathrm{d}t, \tag{3.2.1}$$

subject to a constraint on its size and a constraint that it is orthogonal to previous weight functions

$$\int_0^T \widehat{\xi}_r(t)\widehat{\xi}_r(t)\mathrm{d}t = 1 \text{ and } \int_0^T \widehat{\xi}_r(t)\widehat{\xi}_m(t)\mathrm{d}t = 0 \text{ for } m < r. \tag{3.2.2}$$

Each FPC is a solution to the *functional* eigenequation

$$\int_0^T \hat{v}(s, t)\widehat{\xi}(t)\mathrm{d}t = \widehat{\rho}\widehat{\xi}(s), \tag{3.2.3}$$

where $\widehat{\rho}$ is an eigenvalue that represents the amount of variance explained by the FPC. The first FPC is the solution to Eq. (3.2.3) (called an *eigenfunction*) with the largest eigenvalue and explains the most variance in the data. The variance explained by each successive FPC declines.

Usually, a small number of FPCs capture a large amount of variance in the data, so only the first few are retained. Rules of thumb for choosing the number, R, of FPCs to retain include: choosing enough FPCs so that the total variance explained exceeds a specified threshold (e.g., 95 or 99%); combining this threshold with a minimum variance explained threshold for each individual FPC [121]; or plotting the eigenvalues against the FPC number (called a *scree plot*) to find the "elbow" where the plot tails off. Statistical model-based approaches for choosing R include: cross-validation or Akaike Information Criterion (AIC) [84, Sect. 2.5] or (Restricted) Likelihood Ratio Tests [121]. The choice of approach will likely depend on the purpose of the analysis. If FPCA is being used as an exploratory tool to extract components that describe a movement, the more ad-hoc rules of thumb might be used. If FPC scores are being used in further modelling (e.g., as predictors of sports performance variable in a regression model or to cluster movement profiles, see examples below), then model-based approaches for choosing R could be considered [38].

Importantly, the FPCs can be used as basis functions to approximate each individual curve, where the FPC scores are the basis coefficients of the linear combination

$$\widehat{x}_i(t) = \bar{x}(t) + \sum_{r=1}^{R} \widehat{f}_{ir}\widehat{\xi}_r(t). \tag{3.2.4}$$

This is a truncated Karhunen-Loéve expansion [62]. The representation becomes more accurate as the number of FPCs, R, increases. The FPCs define an *optimal empirical orthonormal basis*—they satisfy the *orthonormality* constraints in (3.2.2), they are estimated from the data (*empirical*) and explain the most variation possible for any set of R basis functions (*optimal*) [4, 20, 120]. Figure 3.4 shows this basis representation for the GaitRec vGRF data. The data are represented in terms of one, two and three FPCs. Each successive FPC adds variation and "shape" to the reconstruction. The basis function representation helps interpretation of the scores and the FPCs since the weighted sum in Eq. (3.2.4) means we can interpret and visualise the scores and FPCs as perturbations of the mean function. Of course, classical PCA for multivariate data can be applied to continuous biomechanical data, treating the data at each time point as a separate variable [122, 123]. In some situations—in particular, when the data are very smooth and realised on a fine, equally-spaced grid—this may mirror FPCA, producing a set of similar or even identical scores [17], but the basis function interpretation is lost if it is not conceptualised as functional. In multivariate PCA, the loadings, which are

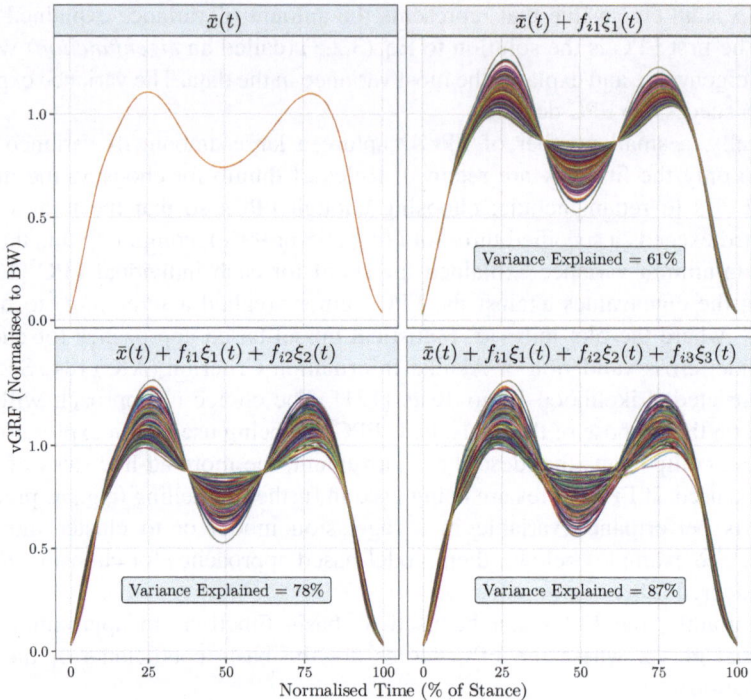

Fig. 3.4 Representation of the vGRF data for the sample of healthy controls from the GaitRec dataset using the sample mean function and a weighted sum of one (top right), two (bottom left) and three (bottom right) estimated FPCs. The top left shows the mean function before any weighted sum of FPCs is added

analogous to the FPCs, do not have any time-dependent structure (or ordering of the dimensions). In addition, viewing the FPCs as smooth functions allows smoothing (or regularisation) to be naturally incorporated into FPCA, which often aids interpretation or improves statistical performance [2, 17, 84, 124].

It should be noted, that like the sample mean and covariance, the FPCs are (functional) statistics that are being estimated from a finite sample of data and hence subject to sampling variability. The extent they would, in theory, vary from sample to sample depends on a number of factors, e.g., the sample size, smoothness and covariance structure of the curves. They should be regarded with the same caution as other quantities that are estimated from the data, particularly in small samples as is often the case in, e.g., elite sports research. In some instances, cross-validation or bootstrapping could be employed in an attempt to understand the uncertainty in the estimated FPCs.

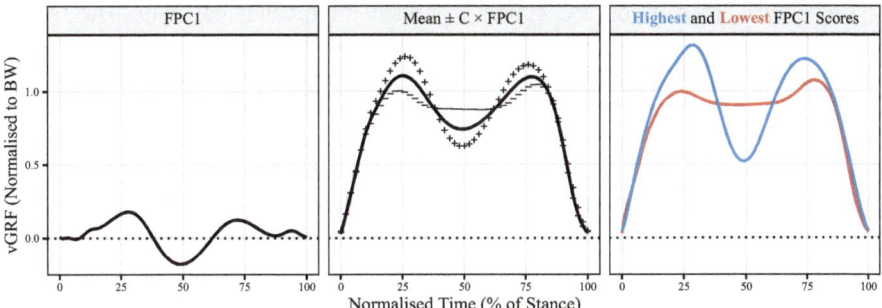

Fig. 3.5 Different options for visualising FPCA demonstrated on FPC1 from the analysis of the vGRF data for the sample of healthy controls from the GaitRec dataset. **Left**: FPC1 plotted as function. **Middle**: The mean function (solid line) with a positive (+) and negative (−) multiple of FPC1 added to it. **Right**: The functions in the dataset with the highest (blue) and lowest (red) FPC1 scores. **Note**: The value of C is chosen to be twice the standard deviation of the associated FPC scores

3.2.2 Uses of FPCA in Biomechanics Research

Both the FPCs and FPC scores can be used to draw insights from biomechanical data. Each FPC has a clear biomechanical interpretation and they lend themselves to intuitive types of visualisation [27, 46]. When applied to biomechanical data, they can be used to summarise and visualise the main sources of variability characterising a movement. This is sometimes the sole motivation for using FPCA [2, 125]. Figure 3.5 displays the first FPC from the GaitRec data. FPC1 is shown in the left-hand plot. It has two positive peaks at about 25 and 75% of the gait cycle, and a negative dip in the middle at 50%. It is capturing the negative dependence between peak heights and dip height that we saw on examining $\hat{v}(s, t)$ in Fig. 3.1. In the middle plot, we show FPC1 as perturbations of the mean function. We have added a positive and negative multiple of FPC1 to the mean function to understand how a positive and negative score on FPC1 "shifts" the mean function. A positive score means increased peak heights and a decreased dip height, whereas a negative score means the opposite, giving a "flatter" curve. The value of the constant, C, multiplied by FPC1 could be chosen as any value within reason. We have chosen C to be twice the standard deviation of the FPC1 scores, which is a default choice in the **fda** R package [118]. On the right, we show the curves from the dataset that had the highest and lowest FPC1 score—these are the extremes of the curves typified in the middle plot.

More often, the resultant FPC scores are used in further analysis. Conventional statistical techniques can be applied to the vectors of FPC scores instead of the functions, hence we say that FPCA achieves "dimension reduction" [62, 126]. For example, FPC scores have been used in clustering [57], discriminant analysis [27] and as dependent variables [60] or independent variables [28] in linear regression models. Some examples are given below.

Liebl et al. [57] used FPC scores to cluster biomechanical data. The overall aim of their study was to compare ankle-plantarflexion strength between rearfoot and forefoot runners. Traditional methods for classification of rearfoot and forefoot footfall patterns suffer from objectivity and reliability issues, and FDA provides a framework in which information on the dynamic footfall pattern can be comprehensively captured. The authors applied FPCA to saggital ankle moment curves and then performed a cluster analysis using the FPC scores to identify footfall patterns. The cluster analysis was performed on data from subjects running barefoot and shod separately. In both cases, it identified clusters of forefoot and rearfoot runners, as defined by traditional metrics. The analysis also identified subjects who switched their footfall pattern upon switching between shod and barefoot running. The clusters were used to test whether runners with different footfall patterns differ in their plantarflexion strength. Plantarflexion strength was significantly higher in the forefoot group even after adjusting for gender and different training levels.

Whereas clustering is an *unsupervised* technique that aims to identify unknown groups, FPC scores can also be used to explore the association of functional observations with *known* groupings in the data. Discriminant analysis has been used to classify group membership using FPC scores. Ryan et al. [27] used scores from FPCA of children's joint angles during the vertical jump in a discriminant analysis to classify the developmental stage of a child's jump performance. They identified FPCs that were important for classifying developmental stages and thus patterns of movement associated with developmental trends. Wu et al. [28] used FPCA scores as predictors in a linear mixed effects model to predict fatigue (a continuous outcome) of recreational athletes. Applying FPCA to the concentric phase of the countermovement jump (CMJ) force-time profile after high-intensity training sessions, they used the scores to predict the fatigue status (in terms of peak relative CMJ force) 6 and 48 hours in advance.

Discriminant analysis uses group as a dependent variable with the FPC scores as independent variables, but the scores can also be modelled as the dependent variable in a regression model. In this case, the group can be included as a categorical independent variable (possibly along with other covariates), and used to examine differences between groups on movement characteristics identified by FPCA. Prosser et al. [56] used this approach to distinguish between muscle activity patterns of children with cerebral palsy and typical development. Using surface EMG collected on 8 muscles bilaterally, they used the continuous wavelet transform (CWT) to obtain a time-frequency pattern for each muscle and performed FPCA on the resulting instantaneous mean frequency (IMNF) curves. FPC scores differed between the two groups on each of the muscles, reflecting that the cerebral palsy group had higher IMNF resulting from altered patterns of muscle unit firing and motor unit recruitment. Donoghue et al. [60] performed FPCA on joint angles of runners with a history of chronic Achilles tendon (AT) injuries and a group of controls captured while running on a treadmill. The AT group ran with and without orthoses, and their FPC scores were compared between the two conditions and also with the control group to understand chronic AT injury mechanisms and how they are affected by the use of orthoses. Differences in FPC scores between the AT and control groups were consistent with previous discrete point analyses but also provided additional information. However, it was FPCA applied separately to each of the individual groups that revealed especially useful information. The control group showed distinct patterns of variability in comparison to the AT group; this motivated further work on this topic [24].

Use of FPCA scores to distinguish between movement patterns of groups has been successful in a biomechanical context but it is important to note its associated caveats. Testing differences between average group FPC scores using a standard linear model framework (i.e., ANOVA or t-test) has drawbacks associated with multiple testing. When there are multiple FPCs on which to test for differences in scores (often between 3 and 5), interpreting the results to report a single difference across a whole movement can be challenging. When FPCA is applied separately to multiple kinetic or kinematic variables, the number of tests increases and interpretation becomes even more difficult. As an alternative, obvious sources of variability between groups could be accounted for with a model and FPCA could be used to explain the remaining variability [20, 125]. For example, Prosser et al. [56] extracted 4 FPCs from the IMNF curves of 16 muscles leading to 64 comparisons. Each difference in FPC scores was statistically significant and indicated a difference in the same direction between the groups at different points in the cycle. Even if problems with Type-I error are corrected, the large number of test results can be challenging to interpret and report collectively. A functional linear model (FLM) would provide a more parsimonious approach, allowing a direct comparison of the mean functions of both groups. FPCA could have subsequently been used to explore the variation in the functional residuals after the group effect was accounted for. We should also note that some FLM approaches model basis coefficients (such as FPC scores) directly, but circumvent the aforementioned difficulties by "transforming back" to do inference and interpretation on the functional scale [22, 81, 127].

The FLM allows comparison of group mean functions, and testing the average difference in FPC scores accomplishes a similar goal. However, comparisons of *variability* between different groups may also be of interest in studies of human movement [24, 128]. For example, increased kinematic variability may indicate good performance or reduced injury risk, as the body is not being loaded repeatedly in the same way on the same structures [24, 129]. Extraction of FPCs for different groups separately is one way to explore this [60]. This approach yields group-specific FPCs that reveal the main sources of variability within a group, but direct comparisons cannot be made between groups [24]. Common functional principal component analysis (CFPCA) [130], the functional analogue of the common principal component analysis [131], was adapted to biomechanical data by Coffey et al. [24] to address this shortcoming. CFPCA assumes that the eigenfunctions of each group's covariance function (i.e., the FPCs) are common across groups, but their relative importance (i.e., the variance that they explain) can vary between groups— this can identify differences between the variance structures of several groups [24]. Coffey et al. [24] applied CFPCA to the AT data from [60] to make comparisons of variability between the AT and control groups based on the relative importance of the common FPCs. CFPCA identified the particular phase of the movement in which variation differed between the groups. A similar approach, in the field of motor learning research, is that of Backenroth et al. [128], who modelled the *variance* of FPCA scores using mixed-effects models. To investigate whether reduction in motion variability in healthy subjects is associated with improvement of motor skill, they studied hand trajectories of repeated reaching motions by subjects to specified targets using FDA. After using functional regression techniques to model average reaching motions, they decomposed the residual variation using FPCA. Similar to CFPCA, they assumed a common set of eigenfunctions (FPCs) for the set of curves, but allowed the variance of the FPCA scores to depend on covariates and random effect terms, exploring the relationship between movement variability and scalar covariates, while accounting for subject-specific effects.

3.2.3   Extensions of FPCA and Future Directions

Standard FPCA [4] is designed for samples of independent functional data [i.e., "first-generation functional data", 62], but does not account for the dependence structure induced by repeated functional observations from the same individual or due to other groupings in the data. In these instances, FPCA can be applied to the combined sample of data, and the dependence structure accounted for post-hoc (e.g., using a scalar mixed effects model for the scores). However, this does not explicitly separate the within and between subject variation in the FPCA step, and the representation in Eq. (3.2.4) assumes independence. Coffey et al. [24] also extended CFPCA to deal with dependent data (e.g., when the same subject is measured under different conditions). CFPCA for dependent data provides a means of quantifying how variability in movement patterns differs under different conditions and across dependent groups in repeated-measures designs, which are fundamental in biomechanics and human movement research. Despite this, CFPCA for dependent groups has seen limited uptake within human movement biomechanics, in part perhaps because an extensive software implementation (e.g., an R package) with associated documentation (e.g., a "how to use" vignette/ tutorial paper) is lacking.

Another approach, that is particularly exciting, is multilevel FPCA (ml-FPCA) [34]. ml-FPCA was first suggested as a possible solution for modelling dependent biomechanical data by Escabias et al. [132], who analysed children's trunk kinematics while carrying backpacks in a repeated-measures design. Di et al. [34] developed ml-FPCA to deal with functional data that have a multilevel or hierarchical structure. Their work was motivated by the sleep heart health study (SHHS), where electroencephalogram (EEG) data, which present naturally as curves, were measured at multiple hospital visits in a longitudinal study. Each EEG profile was modelled as a smooth function, and each visit provided a repeated measure of that function. ml-FPCA was then used to extract FPCs that decompose the main modes of variability between and within subjects (between visits) separately, comprehensively characterising these different sources of functional variation. In biomechanics, the ml-FPCA approach would allow all recorded trials of a movement from multiple subjects to be analysed without averaging or violating independence assumptions, and allow variation to be explored at the between-subject and within-subject levels. ml-FPCA has been generalised to more complex designs with additional levels of grouping [35, 133] (e.g., multiple trials within multiple sessions for each subject). Recently, Matabuena et al. [134] demonstrated how the three-level extension of ml-FPCA [35] can be used to characterise functional variability in runners' knee kinematics between different training sessions. Given that standard FPCA has made a significant impact as a tool for exploring variation in biomechanics and human movement research to date, these new developments, which appropriately account for the complex dependence structures that are commonly encountered in large-scale biomechanical datasets (e.g., GaitRec [5] or Gutenburg [13]), hold significant promise.

Bibliographic Notes

- The GaitRec FPCA example, in particular Fig. 3.5, first appeared in Edward Gunning's Ph.D. thesis (p. 34). Likewise, some of the text in Sect. 3.2.1 on choosing the number of FPCs appeared in Edward Gunning's Ph.D. thesis (pp. 30–31).
- Sect. 3.1 is a synopsis of Ramsay and Silverman [4, pp. 22–24] and Ramsay et al. [20, pp. 83–86].
- The descriptions of the functional boxplot are based on the original paper by Sun and Genton [117] and a more recent review by Genton and Sun [112].
- The description of FPCA is based on Ramsay and Silverman [4, pp. 149–151] and Ramsay et al. [20, pp. 100–102].

Chapter 4
Functional Regression Models in Biomechanics

Abstract This chapter gives an overview of functional regression techniques used to model biomechanical data. Regression with a functional response and scalar covariates, i.e., function-on-scalar regression, is the most commonly used technique in the biomechanical literature. We provide a detailed description of function-on-scalar regression, along with a practical demonstration, comparing vertical ground reaction force functions between groups with different pathologies in the GaitRec dataset. This chapter also describes scalar-on-function (regression with a scalar response and functional covariate) and function-on-function (both response and covariates are functions) regression models and reviews their applications to biomechanical data.

Keywords Functional regression · Function-on-scalar · Scalar-on-function · Function-on-function

4.1 Overview

Functional regression is "the study of associations between variables, when one or more of them are functional" [52, p. 5325]. The dependent (response) variable, one or more of the independent variables (also called predictor variables, covariates or regressors), or both dependent and independent variables can be functions. In biomechanics and human movement research, functional regression models can be used to answer questions such as "How do walking speed, age and gender collectively affect gait patterns?" [64], "Can we predict the onset of fatigue using functional ground reaction force data from the countermovement jump?" [28] and "Can the knee angle function be predicted from the hip angle function during gait?" [20]. To date, *function-on-scalar regression*, where a functional response variable $y(t)$ is regressed on scalar covariates, has received the most attention in biomechanics and human movement applications. Therefore, we will first focus on models of this type, before providing a short description of scalar-on-function and function-on-function regression in the context of biomechanics and human movement research.

© The Author(s), under exclusive license to Springer Nature Switzerland AG 2024   39
E. Gunning et al., *Functional Data Analysis in Biomechanics*,
SpringerBriefs in Statistics, https://doi.org/10.1007/978-3-031-68862-1_4

4.2 Function-on-Scalar Regression

4.2.1 Model Description

For a sample of functional data $y_1(t), \ldots, y_N(t)$ on the time domain[1] $[0, T]$ with associated scalar covariates $x_{ip}, i = 1, \ldots, N$ and $p = 1, \ldots, P$, a function-on-scalar linear[2] regression model is typically written as

$$y_i(t) = \beta_0(t) + \sum_{p=1}^{P} x_{ip}\beta_p(t) + \epsilon_i(t), \qquad (4.2.1)$$

where $\beta_0(t)$ is the intercept function (and often represents the overall mean function), $\beta_1(t), \ldots, \beta_P(t)$ are the regression coefficient *functions* for the covariates $x_1, \ldots x_P$, and $\epsilon_i(t)$ are independent zero-mean random error *functions* with covariance function $C(s, t)$.

Model (4.2.1) resembles a standard multivariable linear regression model, except that the parameters are functions rather than scalars. The regression coefficient functions $\beta_1(t), \ldots, \beta_P(t)$ quantify the linear effects of the scalar covariates $x_1, \ldots x_P$ on the functional response $y(t)$ over the whole time domain $[0, T]$, or more intuitively, how they influence its "expected level and shape" [54, p. 346]. When scalar covariates are coded to represent factor (or group) levels, it is often referred to as a functional analysis of variance (FANOVA), because it is a standard ANOVA (i.e., a comparison of group means) at each point $t \in [0, T]$ [4, 22]. However, function-on-scalar linear regression is more general because it allows both dummy coded (e.g., to represent injury status) and continuous (e.g., walking speed) covariates to influence the functional response.

4.2.2 Estimation

Because Eq. (4.2.1) is a standard multivariable regression at every $t \in [0, T]$, the regression coefficient functions $\beta_0(t), \ldots, \beta_P(t)$ can be estimated pointwise by least squares [136, 137]. First, separate (scalar) linear regression models are fitted to the (smoothed or unsmoothed) functional response at discrete points along the domain by ordinary least squares (OLS). Then, the estimated regression coefficients

---

[1] As motivated by applications in human movement biomechanics, we introduce functional regression for functions defined on a temporal domain. However, these tools can, of course, be applied to functional data that vary over other continua (e.g., space, frequency).

[2] We describe models where the dependent variables are *linearly* related to the independent variables, but note that more flexible, smooth relationships are possible in the functional *additive* mixed model framework of Scheipl et al. [135].

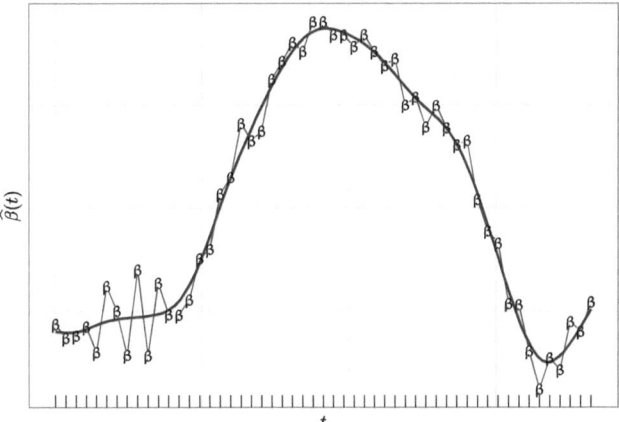

Fig. 4.1 Two-step estimation of a function-on-scalar regression coefficient function. The β represent scalar regression coefficients estimated by fitting linear regression models at points along the time domain, indexed by the rugs (|). The regression coefficient function (dark red line) is constructed by smoothing these pointwise estimates. **Note:** The estimate was obtained by fitting a model to the CanadianWeather data from the **fda** R package using the fosr2s() function in the **refund** R package

at each point are interpolated or smoothed (e.g., using a B-spline basis expansion and roughness penalty) to produce the estimated regression coefficient functions. Benefits of smoothing the regression coefficient function estimates include increased visual interpretability and improved estimation accuracy [22, 136]. This straightforward two-step approach to regression coefficient function estimation is shown in Fig. 4.1.

When the smoothed functional response is represented by a basis function expansion, as described in Chap. 2, it is more natural to express the regression coefficient functions, and hence the least-squares criterion, in terms of basis function expansions too. This reduces the problem to estimating the basis function coefficients of the regression coefficient functions by minimising a single (integrated) least squares criterion. Penalties, typically on the integrated squared second derivative of each regression coefficient function, can be added to the OLS criterion to ensure that the estimates are smooth. The smoothing parameter(s) can be chosen by cross-validation, leaving one function out at a time ("leave-one-function-out cross-validation"—LOFO-CV) [4, 138]. This approach, using penalised least-squares estimation and a basis function expansion for both the functional response and regression coefficient functions, is called "Penalised Ordinary Least Squares" (P-OLS) [138] and it is described extensively by Ramsay and Silverman [4, Chap. 14, pp. 223–246]. It is designed for dense and relatively smooth functional data, where the functional response is represented in terms of a basis function expansion.

A possible drawback of P-OLS is that the *within-function correlation* is ignored. The correlation of $\epsilon_i(t)$ over the domain $[0, T]$ (i.e., that each residual is a smooth function rather than just white noise) is not accounted for in the estimation step, and incorporating it may improve estimation [22, 138]. Therefore, Reiss et al. [138] modified P-OLS to use the an estimate of the residual covariance $C(s, t)$ in the estimation of the model parameters. This is a functional version of generalised least squares (a technique for linear model estimation with correlated errors), so they called it "Penalised Generalised Least Squares" (P-GLS). P-OLS and P-GLS estimation performed similarly in Reiss et al.'s [138] simulated examples. However, specifying the error covariance structure in P-GLS allows a separate smoothing parameter to be chosen for each regression coefficient function using restricted maximum likelihood (REML), allowing more flexibility for different covariate effects to have different levels of smoothness. While it is possible to set up a model with multiple smoothing parameters with P-OLS, choosing them is difficult because it requires a multidimensional grid search to minimise LOFO-CV [138]. As a result, a common smoothing parameter for all regression coefficient functions is typically used, which affords less flexibility for covariate effects to vary in smoothness [138].

Two more general and flexible functional regression modelling frameworks provide methods for function-on-scalar regression [127, 139]. The "Functional Additive Mixed Model" (FAMM) framework [54, 135] is part of the wider functional regression framework of Greven and Scheipl [139]. These models are fitted to the functional response in "raw" form, i.e., sampled on a discrete grid with error, rather than smoothed and represented by a basis expansion. Smoothing and model fitting are combined in the same step and uncertainty due to measurement error is preserved [54, p. 361]. These models handle both sparse and irregular, and dense functional data alike [54, 135]. B-spline basis functions are typically used to represent the regression coefficient functions and they are estimated by penalised likelihood methods, i.e., the functional model is formulated as a scalar generalised additive mixed model (GAMM) for estimation and inference [43, 140]. Hence, this approach extends to non-Gaussian (e.g., count or binary) functional responses and it also allows the effects of scalar covariates to be non-linear.[3] Because the noisy measurements are modelled directly, the error is specified as the sum of two components $\epsilon_i(t) + \varepsilon_{it}$, where $\epsilon_i(t)$ is a smooth random error function as in Eq. (4.2.1) and ε_{it} is white noise as in classical linear regression. The smooth component $\epsilon_i(t)$ is estimated within the model using random effects[4] and basis functions so that a smoothed estimate of each individual curve is produced and within-function covariance is captured [141, 142]. However, these models may not be computationally efficient for large datasets, often because jointly estimating each $\epsilon_i(t)$ alongside all of the other parameters in the model becomes computationally challenging as N becomes large [127, 143, 144]. Using a functional principal component (FPC) rather than spline basis expansion for $\epsilon_i(t)$ can help reduce this concern [133, 141, 145]. The "Functional Mixed Model" (FMM) framework of

---

[3] Instead of linear functional effects of a continous covariate $x_p \beta_p(t)$, the effect of x_p on the functional response is captured in a smooth bivariate function $f(x_p, t)$.

[4] Hence, in these models $\epsilon_i(t)$ is often referred to as "curve-specific functional random intercept" or "curve-specific functional random effect" [22, Sect. 5.6, pp. 340–341]).

Morris [127] also provides an extensive collection of tools for function-on-scalar regression. This framework uses a "basis transform" modelling approach, where a basis function expansion (often, but not exclusively, wavelets) that preserves almost all of the information in the raw functional response variable is used [127, 142, 146]. The basis function coefficients are modelled using Bayesian methods, and the parameter estimates from the models fitted to the basis coefficients are combined with the basis functions to produce estimates on the functional scale. Generally, a basis expansion that produces approximately uncorrelated basis coefficients is used, so that each basis coefficient can be modelled separately. This reduces estimation of the full functional regression model into several smaller model fitting tasks (i.e., a "divide-and-conquer" strategy). As a result, this framework is computationally efficient and highly suitable for large datasets. However, it does not handle sparse, irregularly sampled functional data well. Importantly, both FAMM and FMM frameworks allow various types of "functional random effects" to be incorporated, which can be used to account for, e.g., dependence due to repeated measurements of functions; we expand on this point in Chap. 6. A detailed comparison of both frameworks is given by Morris [127].

4.2.3 Applications in Biomechanics

Applications of function-on-scalar regression (or functional ANOVA) models to gait data include understanding how age, walking speed and gender jointly affect kinematic gait curves [64], comparing kinematic gait data of patients with slipped capital femoral epiphysis and healthy controls [65] and assessing the effect of wearing ankle-foot orthoses for children with cerebral palsy [33], among others [147–151]. In jumping applications, they have been used to examine kinematics and kinetics of individuals with anterior cruciate ligament (ACL) injuries [16, 67–69] and movement strategies in individuals with sprained ankles and healthy controls [152]. Functional ANOVA models have been used in sporting applications, to describe the effects of exercise intensity and asymmetry on the pedal force produced during cycling [153] and on barbell velocity profiles in Olympic weightlifting [154].

We demonstrate function-on-scalar regression using the GaitRec dataset, to compare vertical ground reaction force (vGRF) data between healthy controls and patients with orthopaedic impairment in the ankle, knee, hip and calcaneus. We use an averaged vGRF function from the left side of the body for each subject—this is the injured side for the groups with orthopaedic impairment. The data are shown in Fig. 4.2, coloured according to group. The combined plot of group means in the bottom right shows that, on average, healthy controls differ from the other groups at both peaks and at the dip in the middle of the function (at about 25, 50 and 75% of the stance phase, respectively). The ankle and calcaneus groups have a lower average second peak than the hip and knee groups, whose mean curves are almost identical and cannot be distinguished when overlaid on each other.

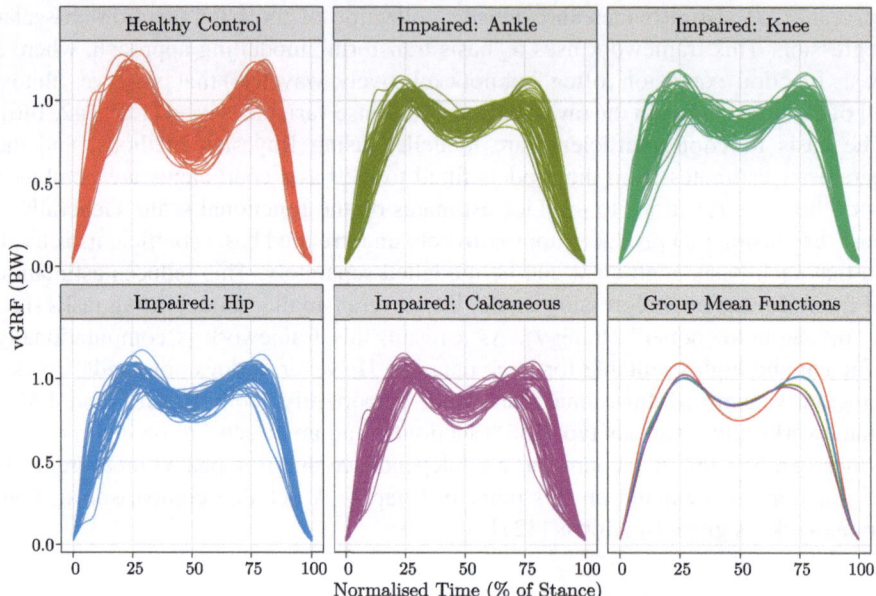

Fig. 4.2 The GaitRec data used in the function-on-scalar regression model. It shows the vGRF from five groups. The bottom right plot shows the group means overlaid on each other

To formalise this comparison of group means, we fit the function-on-scalar regression model

$$y_i(t) = \beta_0(t) + \sum_{p=1}^{5} x_{ip}\beta_p(t) + \epsilon_i(t),$$

where:

- $y_i(t)$ is the vertical ground reaction force function for the ith individual,
- $\beta_0(t)$ is the intercept function,
- $x_{i1}, \ldots, x_{i5}$ are dummy-coded scalar covariates that represent membership of the healthy control and ankle, knee, hip and calcaneus impairment groups,
- $\beta_1(t), \ldots, \beta_5(t)$ are the corresponding regression coefficient functions for scalar covariates $x_{i1}, \ldots, x_{i5}$. We enforce the constraint $\sum_{p=1}^{5} \beta_p(t) = 0$ at each $t \in [0, T]$, so that $\beta_p(t)$ represents the deviation of the pth group from the overall mean function, and
- $\epsilon_i(t)$ is the smooth functional random error term.

We use the `fosr()` function in the **refund** R package [42] to fit the model using the P-GLS method [138]. Figure 4.3 displays the estimated regression coefficient functions $\widehat{\beta}_0(t), \ldots, \widehat{\beta}_5(t)$ and 95% pointwise confidence intervals. The first panel shows the estimated intercept function $\widehat{\beta}_0(t)$, which represents the overall mean

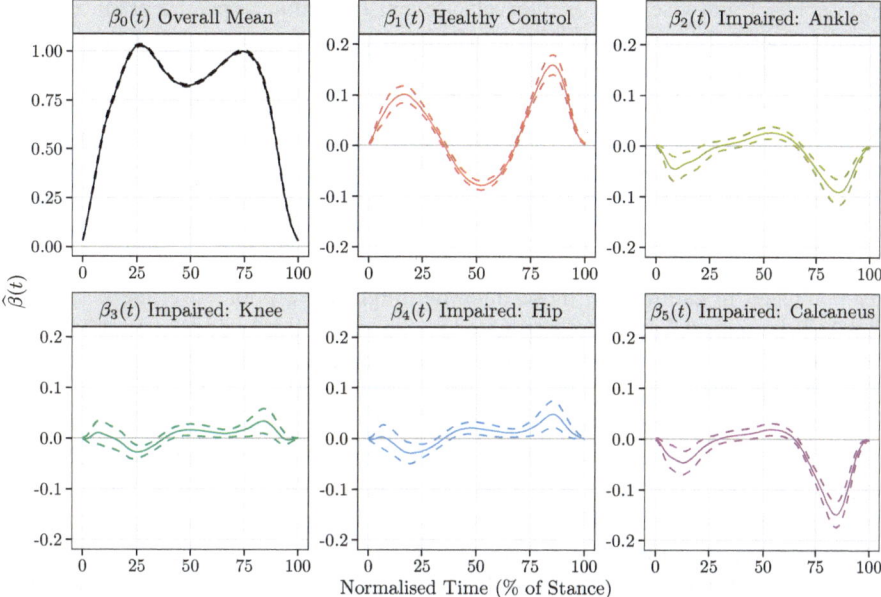

Fig. 4.3 The estimated coefficient functions from the function-on-scalar regression model (solid line) and their associated 95% pointwise confidence intervals (dashed lines). **Note**: The fosr() function in the **refund** R package was used to fit the model using the P-GLS method [138]

function because we have constrained $\widehat{\beta}_1(t), \ldots, \widehat{\beta}_5(t)$ to sum to zero at each $t \in [0, T]$. The healthy control group's regression coefficient function estimate $\widehat{\beta}_1(t)$ represents the largest deviation from the mean, and it reflects the differences between this group and the others seen in Fig. 4.2. The estimated regression coefficient functions for the hip and knee groups ($\widehat{\beta}_2(t)$ and $\widehat{\beta}_3(t)$) are close to zero at all stages of the stance phase, they deviate least from the overall mean. The ankle and calcaneus groups' regression coefficient function estimates ($\widehat{\beta}_4(t)$ and $\widehat{\beta}_5(t)$) both show a negative peak around 75% of the stance phase, reflecting these groups' reduced average second peak seen in Fig. 4.2. In the next section, we review approaches for formally testing and quantifying uncertainty in the estimated regression coefficient functions.

4.2.4 Uncertainty Quantification and Inference

After estimation of a function-on-scalar regression model, constructing confidence intervals or hypothesis tests for the functional coefficients is often of interest (e.g., constructing a confidence interval for $\beta_p(t)$ testing whether some $\beta_p(t) = 0$). In this context, it is important to note the distinction between *pointwise* and *simultaneous* approaches. Pointwise tests or intervals are constructed at a specific point, whereas simultaneous tests or intervals are constructed globally to assess functions on the entire time domain $[0, T]$ [54, 63].

Pointwise confidence intervals for functional regression coefficients, such as those shown in Fig. 4.3, can be constructed in a number of ways. For models fitted using ordinary least squares, Ramsay and Silverman [4, Sect. 13.5.1, pp. 239–241] describe how pointwise confidence intervals can be constructed using standard linear model theory and an estimate of $C(s, t)$ from the model residuals (also described by Reiss et al. [138, Sect. 6.1, pp. 14–15]). When the coefficient functions are penalised in estimation, these intervals might have poor coverage because of bias [138], so models that are estimated in the generalised additive model (GAM) framework (e.g., [54, 135, 138, 139]) use bias-corrected pointwise "empirical Bayesian confidence intervals" as proposed by Nychka [155] (and described in [71, 140, 156]). Bauer et al. [54] describe how straightforward bootstrapping techniques can also be used to derive pointwise confidence intervals. Regardless, the coverage properties of pointwise confidence intervals are designed only to hold at a specific point in the domain. Therefore, although they can be useful for a descriptive analysis, they should not be used to make conclusions about a (group of) functional coefficient(s) *globally* [4, 63]. For this purpose, simultaneous confidence bands or tests should be constructed, though many applications in biomechanics and human movement research have not reported whether the intervals they present are pointwise or simultaneous (e.g., [64, 150, 151, 153, 154]). In the case study in Chap. 6, we demonstrate the use of a bootstrap to construct simultaneous confidence bands for a second application of function-on-scalar regression.

For constructing a global hypothesis test of one or more regression coefficient functions in function-on-scalar regression or functional ANOVA models, the F_{max} procedure is commonly used [4, 20, 138, 157]. The procedure starts by calculating an F-statistic function, i.e., a standard F-statistic calculated on the domain $[0, T]$. For our application, we are interested in the effect of orthopaedic impairments (i.e., whether $\beta_1(t) = \cdots = \beta_5(t) = 0$), so the fitted values from our full model $\hat{y}_i(t) = \hat{\beta}_0(t) + \sum_{p=1}^{5} x_{ip}\hat{\beta}_p(t)$ are used to test against a "null model", consisting of just the sample mean function $\bar{y}(t)$. The F-statistic function is given by

$$F(t) = \frac{(\mathrm{SSY}(t) - \mathrm{SSE}(t))/df_r}{\mathrm{SSE}(t)/df_e},$$

where $\mathrm{SSY}(t) = \sum_{i=1}^{N}(y_i(t) - \bar{y}(t))^2$ is the error sum of squares from the null model, $\mathrm{SSE}(t) = \sum_{i=1}^{N}(y_i(t) - \hat{y}_i(t))^2$ is the error sum of squares from the full model, and both are functions on $[0, T]$. The df_e term is the error degrees of freedom for our full model, which is $N-5$ (the total number of functional observations minus the number of linearly independent regression coefficient functions[5,6]). The df_r

---

[5] The intercept function $\beta_0(t)$ is counted as the first regression coefficient function.

[6] Constraining the 5 regression coefficient functions to sum to zero removes one degree of freedom.

term is the difference in the number of linearly independent functional regression coefficients between the full and null models ($5 - 1 = 4$). The pointwise F-statistic function could be used to conduct separate hypothesis tests along the values of $t \in [0, T]$, by comparing $F(t)$ to the $(1 - \alpha)$th critical value from an F_{df_r, df_e} distribution [158]. However, it is clear that conducting such tests at every point in the domain would lead to an inflated Type-I error rate due to the large (infinite) number of possible comparisons.

The F_{max} procedure is therefore used to construct a simultaneous test from $F(t)$, using the test statistic[7] $F_{max} = \max_{t \in [0,T]} F(t)$ [20]. Critical values for the F_{max} statistic are obtained nonparametrically via *permutation*. To construct an approximate distribution for F_{max} under the null hypotheseis that $\beta_1(t) = \cdots = \beta_5(t) = 0$ for all $t \in [0, T]$, the data are permuted many times, randomly shuffling the functional response while leaving the design matrix of predictor variables (in our example, the orthopaedic impairment group labels) intact, and F_{max} recorded for each permutation [20]. The critical value for a significance test of level α is the $(1 - \alpha)$th percentile of the null distribution. If the observed F_{max} exceeds this critical value, it can be concluded that there exists some $t \in [0, T]$ such that at least one of $\beta_1(t), \ldots, \beta_5(t) \neq 0$. To delineate the intervals on which this difference exists, the pointwise F-statistic can be overlaid on the critical value of F_{max}. The results of an F_{max} test for the function-on-scalar regression model for the GaitRec data are shown in Fig. 4.4. The observed F-statistic function exceeds the critical value (dashed red line) at almost every point in the stance phase—the group mean curves are significantly different due to differences throughout the stance phase.

There are many other methods for testing the statistical significance functional regression coefficients, including bootstrap approaches [137], the functional F-type test based on integrated sums of squares [159], and others (see Górecki and Smaga [160, Sect. 2.1] for a review). In applied biomechanics literature, the F_{max} permutation approach to hypothesis testing is also known as statistical nonparametric mapping (SnPM) [161]. The parametric analogue, statistical parametric mapping (SPM) [162], uses Gaussian random field theory to analytically calculate adjusted test-statistic thresholds (or equivalently, adjusted p-values) for simultaneous inference. It is now widely used in biomechanics and human movement research, and has an extensive open-source software implementation[8] [163]. Warmenhoven et al. [58] compared the FDA permutation, SPM and SnPM implementations of the functional t-test for testing differences in average rowing pin-force curves between males and females. The results from all three approaches demonstrated minimal differences, and led to almost identical conclusions, demonstrating their similarity. More recently, Pataky et al. [157] conducted a comparative study using real and sim-

---

[7] This test statistic is chosen because for any value $F^* > 0$, the following two statements are equivalent: $\{F(t) \leq F^*;$ for all $t \in [0, T]\} \equiv \{\max_{t \in [0,T]} F(t) \leq F^*\}$. In other words, when testing our null hypothesis, if we can conclude that our maximum F-statistic has not exceeded some threshold, we can equivalently conclude that the pointwise $F(t)$ has not crossed that threshold at any $t \in [0, T]$.

[8] https://spm1d.org/.

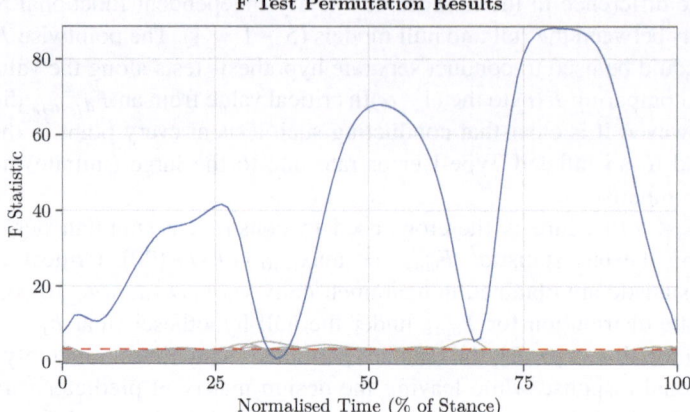

Fig. 4.4 The results of a permutation test (using 500 permutations) for the function-on-scalar regression model fitted to the GaitRec data. The solid blue line is the observed F-statistic, the dashed red line is the 95%th percentile of the approximate null distribution of $F_{max} = \max_{t \in [0,100]} F(t)$ and the grey lines represent the pointwise F-statistics computed for each permutation. **Note**: The `fosr.perm.fit()` function in the **refund** R package was used to conduct the permutation test

ulated sports biomechanics datasets to compare the performance of SPM, the F_{max} permutation approach and two other hypothesis testing techniques—the interval-wise-testing procedure (IWT) and the Benjamini Hochberg (BH) procedure—for identifying specific intervals of the time domain on which significant differences between two mean functions occur. Whereas the F_{max} test is formally a global test for statistical significance across the whole domain, where regions of significance are picked out afterwards (Fig. 4.4), the IWT is a *local* approach that explicitly sets out to find intervals where statistically significant effects occur. The IWP was derived from the Interval Testing Procedure (ITP) [164], which involves representing the functional data being tested by a basis expansion, performing non-parametric multivariate tests on combinations of basis coefficients and calculating an adjusted p-value for each coefficient; it has been used to compare long-term movement impairment in groups of patients who had undergone different treatments for ACL injuries [16, 67]. The IWT generalises the IWP to remove the reliance on a basis expansion and define adjusted p-values for local inference at every point in the domain [165]. Pataky et al. [157] assessed both the Type-I error control and sensitivity to detect differences of all four methods being compared. Their simulation scenarios replicated features present in empirical sports biomechanics datasets (e.g., varying smoothness and variances over the time domain). Overall, the methods performed similarly under many of the scenarios, though specific data characteristics that may influence the methods' performance are detailed. Of note was the similar and robust performance of the SPM and F_{max} approaches on the real and simulated datasets.

4.3 Scalar-on-Function Regression

We describe the most elementary form of scalar-on-function regression where the scalar response variable y_i depends on a single functional covariate $x_i(t)$, for $t \in [0, T]$, $i = 1, ..., N$. The model is

$$y_i = \alpha + \int_0^T \beta(t)x_i(t)\mathrm{d}t + \epsilon_i, \quad \epsilon_i \overset{i.i.d.}{\sim} \mathcal{N}(0, \sigma^2), \tag{4.3.1}$$

where α is the scalar intercept parameter and $\beta(t)$ is the regression coefficient function. For intuition, we should view the coefficient function $\beta(t)$ as a smooth weight function that captures the most important parts of the functional covariate $x_i(t)$ for predicting the scalar response y_i. The Gaussian assumption for ϵ_i means that we are modelling the expected value of the Gaussian response y_i conditional on the function $x_i(t)$. However, the model can be generalised to non-Gaussian responses, such as functional logistic regression for binary outcomes [52, 139].

Sørensen et al. [52] note that in applied contexts, it is generally useful (although an imperfect taxonomy) to view scalar-on-function regression as comprising two main modelling approaches; we follow a similar presentation style here. The first modelling approach is functional principal components regression (FPCR). FPCR involves applying FPCA to $x_i(t)$, extracting the first R FPCs, $\widehat{\xi}_r(t), r = 1, ..., R$, and regressing y_i on the associated scalar FPC scores

$$y_i = \alpha + \sum_{r=1}^R \widehat{f}_{ir}\beta_r + \epsilon_i, \tag{4.3.2}$$

with the scalar regression coefficients β_r estimated using standard multivariable linear regression. The weighted sum $\beta(t) = \sum_{r=1}^R \beta_r \widehat{\xi}_r(t)$ reconstructs the coefficient function.[9] The number of components R controls the smoothness of

---

[9] Implicitly, when we enter scores as predictor variables, we are using the truncated Karhunen-Loéve expansion to represent $x_i(t) - \bar{x}(t) = \sum_{r=1}^R \widehat{f}_{ir}\widehat{\xi}_r(t)$ and also using the FPCs as basis functions to represent $\beta(t) = \sum_{r=1}^R \beta_r \widehat{\xi}_r(t)$. Substituting these into the integral and re-arranging it as follows

$$\int_0^T \beta(t)(x_i(t) - \overline{x}(t))\mathrm{d}t = \int_0^T \underbrace{\sum_{r_1=1}^R \beta_{r_1}\widehat{\xi}_{r_1}(t)}_{\beta(t)} \underbrace{\sum_{r_2=1}^R \widehat{f}_{ir_2}\widehat{\xi}_{r_2}(t)}_{x_i(t)-\overline{x}(t)} \mathrm{d}t$$

$$= \sum_{r_1=1}^R \sum_{r_2=1}^R \beta_{r_1}\widehat{f}_{ir_2} \underbrace{\int_0^T \widehat{\xi}_{r_1}(t)\widehat{\xi}_{r_2}(t)\mathrm{d}t}_{\substack{=1 \text{ if } r_1=r_2 \text{ and } 0 \text{ if } r_1 \neq r_2, \\ \text{because FPCs are orthonormal.}}}$$

$$= \sum_{r=1}^R \beta_r \widehat{f}_{ir}$$

reduces it to the non-functional scalar multivariable regression model (4.3.2).

$\beta(t)$; choosing more components will give a higher resolution. FPCR is a tractable approach—it is based upon the notion that because the FPCs provide a parsimonious representation of $x(t)$, they should also be useful for expressing its relationship with y (though this need not be the case) [52, 139] [126, pp. 221–223]. In addition, it does not require any sophisticated tools, and can be implemented using familiar linear regression software (e.g., lm() in R), by inputting the FPC scores as scalar predictor variables. However, as we show in the case study in Chap. 5, the estimate of $\beta(t)$ is highly dependent on the number of FPCs used, which motivates a more flexible approach that allows finer control in regularising this estimate.

The other, more flexible, approach involves using a general basis expansion and a roughness penalty for $\beta(t)$. By expanding $\beta(t)$ in terms of K_β basis functions $\{\phi_k(t)\}_{k=1}^{K_\beta}$ (e.g., Fourier or B-spline) such that $\beta(t) = \sum_{k=1}^{K_\beta} b_k \phi_k(t)$, we can minimise the penalised least squares criterion

$$\text{PENSSE}(\alpha, \beta) = \sum_{i=1}^{N} \left(y_i - \alpha - \int_0^T x_i(t)\beta(t)dt \right)^2 + \lambda \text{PEN}(\beta(t)), \qquad (4.3.3)$$

where $\text{PEN}(\beta(t))$ is a general regularisation penalty on the regression coefficient function [4, p. 266][53]. In many cases, the integrated squared second derivative of $\beta(t)$ is penalised to enforce smoothness (as discussed earlier in this chapter and in Chap. 2), but other techniques that focus directly on interpretability of $\beta(t)$ rather than smoothness have been proposed [166]. The value of λ can be chosen via the cross-validation and maximum-likelihood approaches described in the context of smoothing individual curves in Chap. 2 (e.g., CV, GCV and REML). Reiss et al. [167, Sect. 2.3, p. 231] review some "hybrid approaches" that combine the FPCR and flexible basis expansion methods. In Chap. 5, we demonstrate a number of implementations of scalar-on-function regression in an application to the GaitRec dataset.

There have been limited applications of scalar-on-function regression in biomechanics. It is more common for functional data to be treated as an outcome, and modelled as a response variable. However, there have been some exceptions. The prediction of fatigue in recreational athletes using FPC scores by Wu et al. [28], noted in Chap. 3, is an application of FPCR. In addition, scalar-on-function logistic regression has been introduced to develop prognostic biomechanical models, classifying individuals with neck [168] and back [169] pain. These prognostic models were fitted using model-based boosting (i.e., the **FDboost** [170] framework), which produced clinically interpretable predictive models from a large number of functional and scalar biomechanical predictor variables. Whereas traditionally the field has treated functional variables as outcomes and employed, e.g., hypothesis tests, it is possible that this work constitutes a shift towards *prediction* from functional biomechanical data in an FDA framework, especially as data collection moves beyond the traditional laboratory experiment environment.

4.4 Function-on-Function Regression

For function-on-function linear regression, model (4.3.1) can be changed to have a functional response $y_i(t)$. The concurrent functional model

$$y_i(t) = \alpha(t) + \beta(t)x_i(t) + \epsilon_i(t), \tag{4.4.1}$$

assumes that the value of $y_i(t)$ only depends on $x_i(t)$ through its value at the "current" time t. In contrast, the *non-concurrent* (or *full* or *total*) model

$$y_i(t) = \alpha(t) + \int_0^T \beta(s, t)x_i(s)\mathrm{d}s + \epsilon_i(t), \tag{4.4.2}$$

allows $y_i(t)$ to be influenced by values of $x_i(t)$ over the whole interval [53]. Typically, the regression coefficient functions are again expanded in terms of basis functions and estimated using penalised least-squares [52]. A type of "hybrid" between the concurrent and non-concurrent models, called the *historical functional linear model* [171], is obtained by modifying the non-concurrent model to only allow the functional covariate to influence "future" values of the functional response

$$y_i(t) = \alpha(t) + \int_{t-\delta}^t \beta(s, t)x_i(s)\mathrm{d}s + \epsilon_i(t), \quad 0 < \delta \le t.$$

The key distinction here is that the upper limit on the integral is the current time t and not the maximum time T, which can be interpreted as a restriction that does not allow us to "look past" the current value of $x(t)$ when trying to predict $y(t)$. The time lag δ indicates how far we can "look back"; this can be the whole covariate function's history if we set $\delta = t$. Ramsay and Silverman [47] and Malfait and Ramsay [171] used this approach to capture a "feedforward" effect of EMG activity on kinematic lip data, where the historical model was preferred to the concurrent model because it accounted for an anticipated delay (or lag) between neural excitation observed through the EMG measurements and the corresponding muscle movements in the kinematic data. We posit that such a model may be very useful in biomechanical applications.

Function-on-function regression models can be used to study the relationship between different kinematic and kinetic variables collected during a movement (e.g., predicting knee angle from hip angle using the concurrent model in Ramsay et al. [20, Sect. 10.2.3, pp. 158–162]). Importantly, rather than model the relationship between two different functional variables, function-on-function regression also enables the relationship between a function and its own derivatives to be modelled, to uncover "dynamic" relationships (we will mention this approach in Chap. 6).

Bibliographic Notes

- Text and examples in this chapter first appeared in Chap. 2 of Edward Gunning's Ph.D. thesis [55, pp. 37–45]. In particular, versions of Figs. 4.1, 4.2 and 4.3 appeared on p. 39, p. 43 and p. 45 of the thesis, respectively.
- There are full chapters in Ramsay and Silverman [4] dedicated to function-on-scalar regression (Chap. 13, pp. 223–246), scalar-on-function regression (Chap. 15, pp. 261–278) and function-on-function regression (Chaps. 14 and 16, pp. 247–260 and pp. 279–296).
- Full methodological reviews of general functional regression and scalar-on-function regression are provided by Morris [22] and Reiss et al. [167], respectively.
- Practical aspects of functional regression in other fields of application are reviewed by Sørensen et al. [52], Bauer et al. [54] and Coffey and Hinde [53].

Chapter 5
Case Study: The GaitRec Data

Abstract The aim of this chapter is to bring together the concepts and applications reviewed and described in Chaps. 2–4 by means of a practical case study on the large-scale, publicly-available GaitRec biomechanics dataset. The focus of this chapter is on practical implementation, so equations and mathematical notation are kept to a minimum, and the R packages and commands used to perform the analysis are noted. All code needed to reproduce the case study is available at GitHub (https://github.com/FAST-ULxNUIG/SpringerBriefs).

Keywords Data analysis · Ground reaction force · Functional principal components analysis · Functional regression

5.1 Overview

5.1.1 Data Description

For this case study, we use the GaitRec dataset [5], which was introduced in Chap. 1 and used to demonstrate techniques in subsequent chapters. This dataset is described by Horsak et al. [5] and is freely available for download from the corresponding data repository.[1] In the accompanying code for this chapter, we have written a script that downloads the dataset and reads it into R.

For an in-depth, technical description of the data collection and processing, we recommend reading the GaitRec data descriptor [5]; we provide a less technical overview in this section. The dataset contains bilateral ground reaction force (GRF) and centre of pressure (COP) measurements recorded during walking trials using force plates in a clinical gait lab setting. We focus on the GRF measurements, and initially work with all three force components (i.e., the vertical, anterior-posterior and medio-lateral components). Walking trials from more than 2000 patients with musculoskeletal impairments and over 200 healthy controls were

---

[1] https://doi.org/10.6084/m9.figshare.c.4788012.v1.

© The Author(s), under exclusive license to Springer Nature Switzerland AG 2024
E. Gunning et al., *Functional Data Analysis in Biomechanics*,
SpringerBriefs in Statistics, https://doi.org/10.1007/978-3-031-68862-1_5

measured. Within a session, multiple walking trials are available for each individual, and some individuals were recorded on more than one session. For example, healthy controls walked at different speeds (slow, self-selected and fast), and the impaired patients "walked either barefoot, with their orthopaedic or normal shoes, and with or without orthopaedic insoles" [5, p. 2]. Therefore, metadata of each subject's characteristics (e.g., age, weight, height, orthopaedic impairment label/ healthy control) and about the settings of each session (e.g., speed, shod condition) accompany the biomechanical data, along with an indicator for each trial (see Table 3 of [5]). In Sects. 5.1.2 and 5.3.2, we describe how we narrow this vast dataset down into smaller subsets that are suitable for a short case study.

The raw GRF measurements are publicly available at the data repository. However, the authors also provide data that are processed according to their laboratory's internal standards. In particular, the processed GRF data are:

- Low-pass filtered using a 2nd-order Butterworth filter [9]. The cut-off frequency of 20 Hz was chosen based on previous literature,
- Linearly time normalised to the interval [0, 100]% so that 0 represents the start of the stance phase and 100% the end,
- Normalised by the participants body weight (BW) so that the force represents a "proportion of body weight").

We use the processed data in this case study to maintain the standards proposed by the GaitRec authors. Consequently, we do not have to perform the linear time normalisation ourselves and we do not have to heavily re-smooth the data because they have already been filtered (covered in Sect. 5.2.1). In short, we can say that observations in the data represent:

Measurements of the vertical, anterior-posterior and medio-lateral ground reaction force components, normalised to body weight and sampled on the normalised time grid 0, 1, ..., 100, where 0(%) represents the start of the stance phase (i.e, foot strike on the force platform) and 100(%) represents the end of the stance phase (i.e, toe-off the force platform).

5.1.2 Scope and Limitations

The scope and structure of the GaitRec data is vast and complex and facilitates several types of statistical analyses (e.g., between subjects, within subjects between sessions or conditions, longitudinal analyses). We choose to narrow the scope to make this case study more comprehensible, by working with a standardised subset of the data that has been provided by the authors for training machine learning models (see TRAIN_BALANCED in [5]). In particular, for each individual, only data from their initial measurement session are included. In addition, only sessions which contain at least five bilateral walking trials are used. Summary characteristics of the participants in this subset are presented in Table 5.1. In this chapter, we first use data from the healthy controls to study the relationship between the vertical GRF curves

Table 5.1 Summary characteristics of the subset of GaitRec data used in this case study. For more information on the participants in this subset, see TRAIN_BALANCED in Horsak et al. [5]

		Mean	Std. Dev.
Age (years)		40.8	12.4
Body mass (kg)		81.0	16.7
		N	(%)
Sex	Female	195	26.9
	Male	530	73.1
Impairment class	Healthy control	145	20.0
	Ankle	145	20.0
	Knee	145	20.0
	Hip	145	20.0
	Calcaneus	145	20.0

and the maximum anterior-posterior GRF (Sects. 5.3.2.1 and 5.4.1). We then use data from all participants to study differences in the anterior-posterior GRF curves between the different impairment classes (Sects. 5.3.2.2 and 5.4.2).

From a statistical modelling perspective, we also narrow the scope of the case study. Although we describe the initial processing and visualisation for the entire dataset, we use session-averaged curves when applying FDA techniques. Of course, in general, it is preferable to use data from individual trials directly and implement more sophisticated multilevel FDA approaches that are noted as pertinent future directions in Chap. 6. In a similar vein, we perform analyses of each force component separately (i.e., *univariately*) but, in general, would advocate for a single integrated *multivariate* FDA approach.

5.1.3 Software

All analyses are performed in the R programming language [172] version 4.1.2. We primarily use the **fda** [118] and **refund** [42] R packages and we note within the text which functions are used.[2] The code for all analyses outlined in this chapter is contained in R and Quarto notebooks, available at https://github.com/FAST-ULxNUIG/SpringerBriefs.

5.2 Preparation for Analysis

5.2.1 Basis Expansion

As noted in Chap. 2, there is generally no need to re-smooth data when they are already smooth because they have been filtered using conventional biomechanical

---

[2] Unless otherwise stated, it should be assumed that commands belong to the **fda** package.

Fig. 5.1 A boxplot
displaying the approximation
error (square root of the SSE)
for each individual curve
given by a basis expansion
using K basis functions, for
values of K from 15 and 80

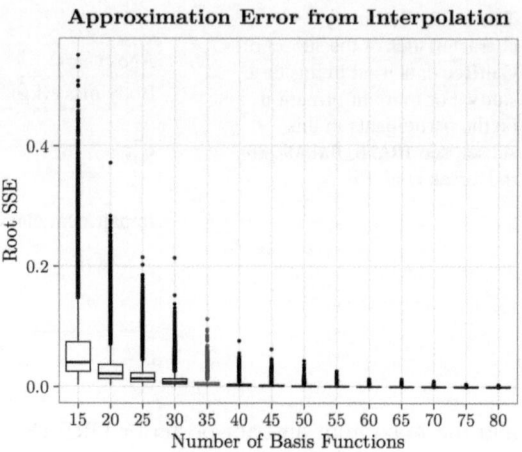

techniques. However, basis function methodologies can still be used to convert each
vector of discrete measurements to a smooth function. In this setting, we are not
concerned with balancing smoothness and fit to the data; our primary objective is
choosing a basis that can interpolate the discrete measurements almost perfectly.
Of course, using substantially more basis functions than we actually need would
be computationally inefficient as it would increase the dimensionality of the basis
coefficient matrix being stored and used in subsequent analysis.

For the reasons outlined in Chap. 2, we choose a cubic B-spline basis. We then
take a pragmatic approach[3] to choosing K, the number of basis functions. That is,
we construct a simple `for` loop to iterate through a number of potential values for K.
On each iteration, we use the `create.bspline.basis()` function to create a cubic
B-spline basis of size K, and we approximate each observation using this basis, estimating the basis coefficients by ordinary least squares with the `smooth.basis()`
function. We record the sum of squared errors (SSE) for each individual curve, as a
measure of the quality of the approximation. Figure 5.1 displays the results of this
procedure. As expected, the approximation error decreases as K increases. Based
on visual inspection, we opt for $K = 35$ basis functions (highlighted in green) as
it appears that the decrease in approximation error gained by increasing K beyond
this point is limited. Figure 5.2 displays a random sample of three curves from the
dataset fitted with our chosen basis of $K = 35$ cubic B-splines, for each of the three
force components.

---

[3] This approach was also taken in the thesis of Gunning [55, p. 70] to represent a large kinematic
dataset and is closely related to the idea of a "near-lossless basis expansion" [22, 127, 142].

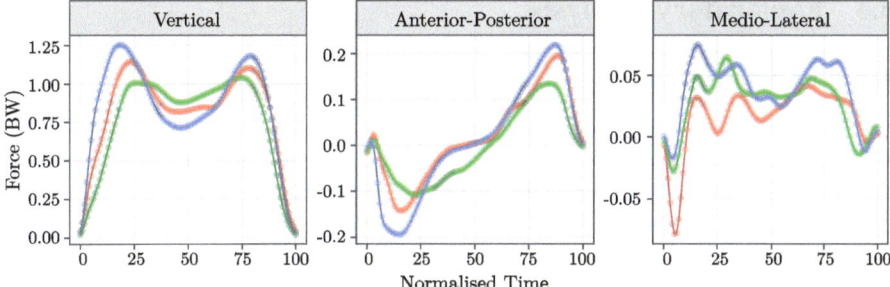

Fig. 5.2 Three randomly chosen observations from the GaitRec dataset. The sampled discrete values are shown as semi-transparent points and the fitted functions using $K = 35$ B-spline basis functions are overlaid as solid lines

5.2.2 Registration

We do not register the data to keep the case study brief. However, registration could be applied, because even in the sample of three curves in Fig. 5.2, there appears to be some temporal misalignment of features. If landmarks are clearly identifiable in every curve then landmark registration could be applied using the `landmarkreg()` function. Inspecting the curves in Fig. 5.2, the negative and positive peaks in the anterior-posterior component appear as potentially useful candidates for this task. These also represent biomechanically meaningful instances in the stance phase, with the first (negative) peak relating to the maximal "braking" force and the second (positive) peak relating to the maximal propulsive force within a cycle. Alternatively, the continuous registration described in Ramsay and Silverman [4, pp. 138–140] could be applied using the `register.fd()` function.

As practical guidance, as we have three force components measured concurrently during the movement (i.e., multivariate functional data), we advise registering each of the force components using the same warping functions. Hypothetically, this might mean choosing a landmark from the anterior-posterior component that represents a biomechanically meaningful instance in the stance phase, and then using it to register the vertical, anterior-posterior and medio-lateral force components simultaneously. Importantly, this preserves the temporal correlation between the three components [55, p. 108]. We also advise that an effort be made to assess the sensitivity of any results to registration, and warping functions or landmarks be incorporated or presented in further analysis, where possible. Finally, it should also be noted that the linear time normalisation procedure applied by the GaitRec authors is itself a version of registration [5].

5.3   Exploratory Analysis

5.3.1   Graphics

We begin our exploratory analysis of the dataset by constructing functional boxplots
[117] of the three force components using the `boxplot.fd()` function (Fig. 5.3).
The functional median, indicated by the solid black line represents the most typical
curve in the dataset. The purple ribbons indicate the variability of the most central
50% of curves. No outlying curves are identified for any of the three components
(i.e., no individual functions are overlaid in red). However, it cannot be conclusively
stated that atypical curves are not present in this sample. Reasons for this include:

- The variability in this combined sample (i.e., all participants described in
  Table 5.1) might mask outliers within each of the classes (e.g., some might be
  identified if the boxplot were restricted to the healthy controls), or
- Outliers might be multivariate (functional) in nature, and a more sophisticated
  visualisation encompassing all three force components jointly (e.g., [112]) may
  be required to reveal them.

We should also note that the GaitRec authors performed an internal outlier screening
[5]. Nonetheless, the functional boxplot provides a simple and interpretable visual
summary of this kinetic dataset.

5.3.2   Functional Principal Components Analysis

In this section, we apply FPCA separately to two different subsets of the GaitRec
data, and use the resultant scores in a descriptive fashion to highlight the relationships between variables, which we then investigate more formally using functional
regression models in Sect. 5.4. In both cases, we work with the sample mean curve

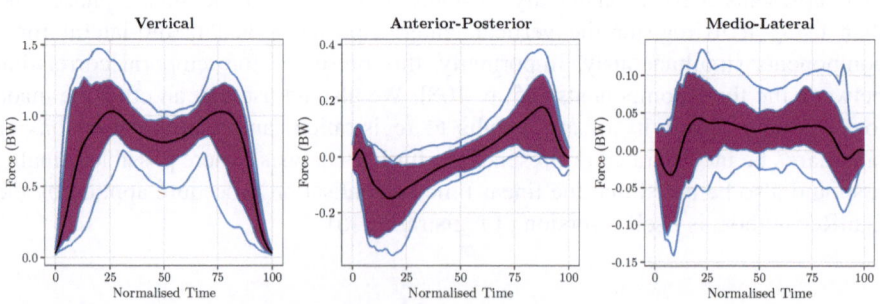

Fig. 5.3 Functional boxplots of the three force components constructed using the `boxplot.fd()`
function

from all trials, calculated on the right and left side separately for each individual. To calculate the mean of a group of curves that are expanded on a given basis, we simply take the mean of each their basis coefficients.[4]

5.3.2.1 Functional Principal Components Analysis 1: Healthy Controls

In this section, we work with the data from the healthy controls (i.e., the HC class [5]) only. So that we have an independent sample, we work with the right side sample mean curves (a paired/ multilevel approach would be needed to account for correlation among bilateral observations from the same individual).

We apply FPCA separately to the vertical and anterior-posterior GRF components, using the `pca.fd()` function. This function takes the functional data that are represented by a basis expansion (i.e., as an `fd` object) and calculates the FPCs directly from the basis representation. By default, the FPCs are represented by the same basis as the data, but any basis can be specified. It also allows a smoothing penalty to be included in the calculation of the FPCs which is often advisable because it enhances estimation accuracy and interpretability of the estimated FPCs. Here, however, both the functional observations and the extracted FPCs appeared smooth, so we did not add any penalty.

In both cases, 5 FPCs explain approximately 90% of the variance (91% for vertical and 89% for anterior-posterior). We display the first three components as perturbations of the mean function in Fig. 5.4. In this visualisation, the '+' curve represents a typical curve that has a positive (or higher-than-average) score on a given FPC, and the '−' curve represents a typical curve that has a negative (or lower-than-average) score on that FPC. For the vertical GRF component, the first FPC resembles that presented in Chap. 3 (a similar sample was used but with the left leg instead of right, and we applied a light registration in Chap. 3, but not here). Generally, an observation with a positive score on this FPC (the '+' curve) is characterised by a higher-than-average first and second peak, and a lower-than-average dip in the middle of the curve. The second FPC seems to represent a shift in the horizontal direction, indicating that it is capturing phase variability that might otherwise be removed through registration. For the anterior-posterior GRF component, a negative score on the first FPC (the '−' curve) enhances the two peaks—the first (negative) peak becomes more negative, the second (positive) peak is increased. Akin to the vertical component, the second FPC seems to capture some phase variation.

As an initial exploration, we examine the cross-correlation between the two sets (i.e., one for each force component) of FPC scores extracted (Fig. 5.5a). There are strong correlations between the first two FPCs from the two force components (−0.81 and −0.82). This is not surprising, since these are complimentary measure-

---

[4] When the group of curves is represented as a single `fd` object, the `mean.fd()` function does exactly this "under the hood".

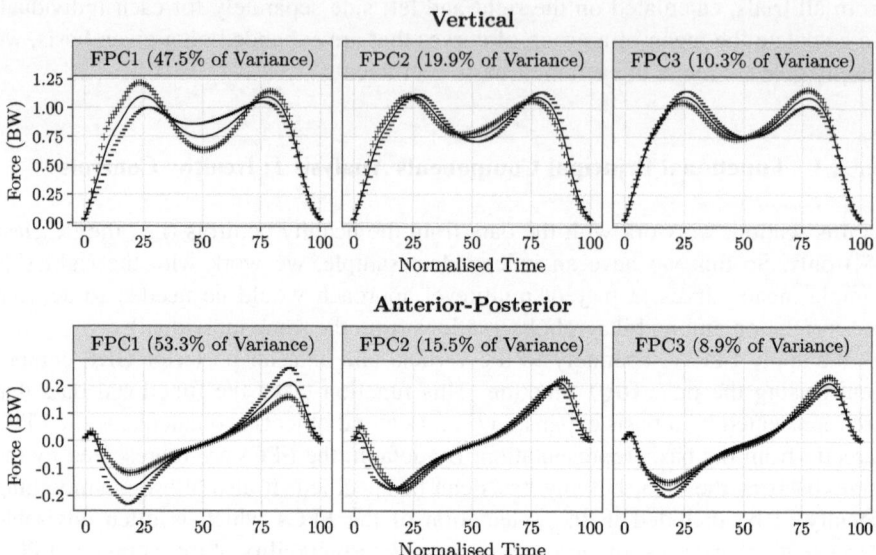

Fig. 5.4 The first three FPCs, shown as perturbations of the mean function, from the FPCA of the sample of healthy controls for the vertical (top panel) and anterior-posterior (bottom panel) GRF components

ments of the same movement so we would expect them to be intrinsically linked. This suggests that, for example, if we were modelling both functional variables as outcomes or predictors in a functional model, it would be advisable to account for the dependence between them using an approach such as multivariate FPCA (mv-FPCA). In fact, Happ and Greven [38] have developed a mv-FPCA algorithm which is specifically based on the cross-correlations among the univariate FPC scores seen in Fig. 5.5a.

For this demonstration, we use the functional data from the vertical GRF component to predict a discrete variable taken from the anterior-posterior GRF component, namely the maximum anterior-posterior force. We calculate the maximum anterior-posterior force by evaluating the anterior-posterior force curves on a grid of $t = 0, 1, \ldots, 100$ to find the global maximum. The most straightforward way to examine this relationship graphically is to plot the FPC scores from our functional variable (vertical force) against our discrete variable of interest (the maximum anterior-posterior force); this visualisation is presented in Fig. 5.5b. We see a moderately-strong, linear relationship between the first vertical FPC score and the maximum anterior-posterior force. In Sect. 5.4, we demonstrate how this relationship can be formally modelled using a scalar-on-function regression model, first by using the FPC scores calculated in this section in a standard multivariable linear regression model, and then using more sophisticated functional regression techniques.

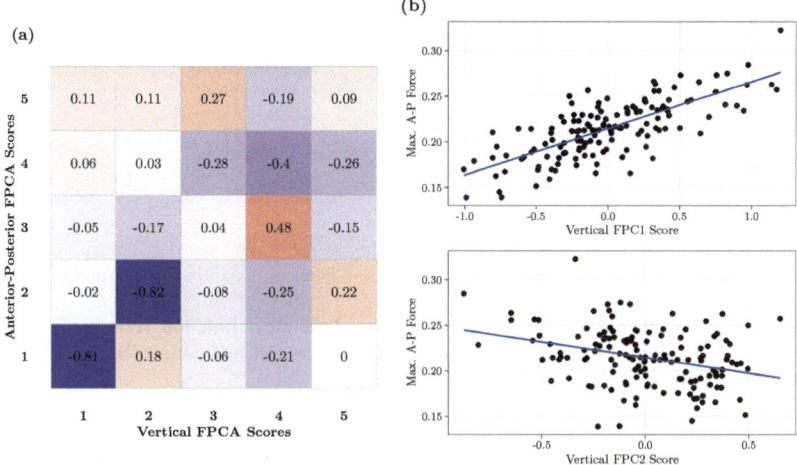

Fig. 5.5 (**a**) The cross-correlations between the extracted vertical (*x*-axis) and anterior-posterior (*y*-axis) FPCA scores. (**b**) A scatterplot of the first (top) and second (bottom) FPC scores from the FPCA of the vertical GRF component against the maximum anterior-posterior force variable

5.3.2.2   Functional Principal Components Analysis 2: Impaired Movement

In our second analysis, we investigate how movement impairment is related to the anterior-posterior GRF component. We work with data from all 725 participants described in Table 5.1. That is, we have data from healthy controls and individuals with orthopaedic impairment in the ankle, knee, hip and calcaneus. For the comparison, we use data from the right side for the healthy controls and individuals with an impairment on both sides, and we use data from the affected side of individuals with an impairment on a single side. As an initial exploratory step, we apply FPCA to the combined set of anterior-posterior GRF curves from all of the groups. Figure 5.6 displays the first three FPCs from this analysis, plotted as perturbations of the mean function. Figure 5.7 displays boxplots of the corresponding FPC scores according to the orthopaedic impairment group. For FPC1, there appears to be a difference between the groups, most notably between the healthy controls and the others. For example, the leftmost boxplot in Fig. 5.7 indicates that the healthy controls appear to have, on average, higher FPC1 scores than the other groups. Mapping this back to the leftmost plot in Fig. 5.6, where the '+' curve indicates a typical observation with a higher-than-average FPC1 score, we can deduce that the healthy controls tend to produce higher braking (i.e., more negative first peak) and propulsive (i.e., more positive second peak) forces, compared to the groups with different pathologies. In Sect. 5.4.2, we demonstrate the use of a function-on-scalar regression model to make the comparison of the anterior-posterior GRF curves between these groups in a more formal way.

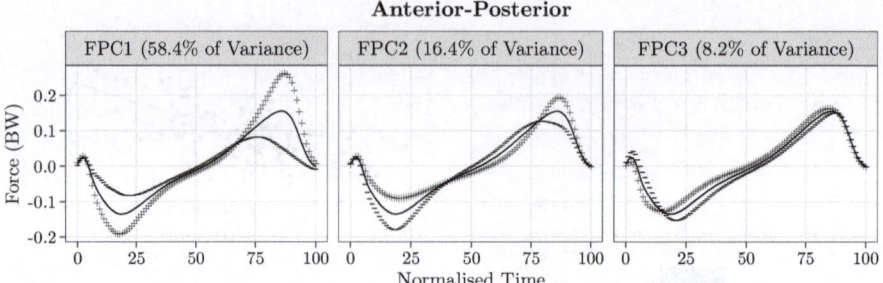

Fig. 5.6 The first three FPCs, shown as perturbations of the mean function, from the FPCA of the anterior-posterior GRF on the dataset containing healthy controls and patients with impairment in the ankle, knee, hip and calcaneus

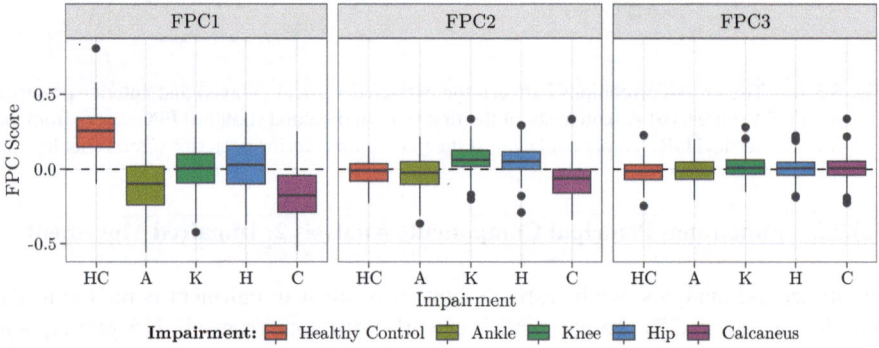

Fig. 5.7 Boxplots of the first three FPC scores from the FPCA of the anterior-posterior GRF on the dataset containing healthy controls and patients with impairment in the ankle, knee, hip and calcaneus

5.4 Functional Regression

5.4.1 Scalar-on-Function Regression: Healthy Controls

In this section, we return to investigating the relationship between the functional vertical GRF variable and the (discrete) maximum anterior-posterior GRF variable, which we examined graphically in Fig. 5.5b. We can formulate the corresponding scalar-on-function regression model as

$$y_i^{\mathrm{AP}} = \alpha + \int_0^{100} x_i^V(t)\beta(t)\mathrm{d}t + \epsilon_i, \quad \epsilon_i \overset{i.i.d.}{\sim} \mathcal{N}(0, \sigma^2),$$

where y_i^{AP} is the maximum anterior-posterior GRF scalar variable for subject i, $x_i^V(t)$ is the vertical GRF function for subject i, and ϵ_i is the random error term.

There are 145 healthy controls in this sample, so i ranges from 1 to 145. Our objective is to estimate the unknown regression coefficient function $\beta(t)$, which weights the vertical GRF curve at different time points to predict the maximum anterior-posterior force.

The first approach we take is functional principal component regression (FPCR), where we use the scalar FPC scores from the FPCA of the vertical GRF variable in Sect. 5.3.2.1 to predict y^{AP} using standard multivariable linear regression. We denote the FPC scores by $\widehat{f}_{ir}^{V}$ to give the linear regression model

$$y_i^{AP} = \alpha + \sum_{r=1}^{R} \widehat{f}_{ir}^{V} \beta_r + \epsilon_i.$$

This is a standard (non-functional) multivariable linear regression model, so we fit it using the lm() function in R. We denote the estimates of $\beta_1, \ldots, \beta_R$ by $\widehat{\beta}_1, \ldots, \widehat{\beta}_R$. As noted in Chap. 4, these estimates from the multivariable linear regression model can be combined with the estimated FPCs from Sect. 5.3.2.1, denoted by $\widehat{\xi}_r^{V}(t)$, to give our estimate of the regression coefficient *function*

$$\widehat{\beta}(t) = \sum_{r=1}^{R} \widehat{\beta}_r \widehat{\xi}_r^{V}(t).$$

Because this estimate is dependent on the number of FPCs used (R), we trial all possible values for R: $1, \ldots, 35$. In this case, 35 is the maximum possible number of FPCs because we have used 35 basis functions to represent the data [4, p. 154]. Figure 5.9a displays a selection of the resulting estimates for $\widehat{\beta}(t)$. As expected, larger values of R produce wigglier estimates of $\beta(t)$. To choose the optimum value of R, we perform a leave-one-out cross-validation (LOO-CV) loop and choose the value of R that produces the lowest average out-of-sample prediction error. This turns out to be $R = 11$ (Fig. 5.8). To avoid data leakage (i.e., curves in the test fold being used to calculate the FPCs and hence in model "training"), estimation of both the FPCs and the regression model is performed on the training fold only, while the test fold is used exclusively for assessing predictions. In other words, we calculate new FPCs for each cross-validation fold.

We now turn to two more refined solutions for fitting the model—the fRegress() function in the **fda** package and the pfr() function in the **refund** package [42]. Both of these implementations represent $\beta(t)$ using a general basis expansion and allow a roughness penalty to be placed on the estimated regression coefficient function. As fRegress() uses the **fda** package's convention, we supply the same basis of 35 cubic B-splines that we used to represent the data, as a basis to represent $\beta(t)$, and we place a roughness penalty on the integrated squared second derivative of $\beta(t)$ to enforce smoothness. The penalty parameter λ then controls the level of smoothness; the effects of varying it over a large range of values are shown in Fig. 5.9b. To choose a suitable value, we again use LOO-CV, this time using the

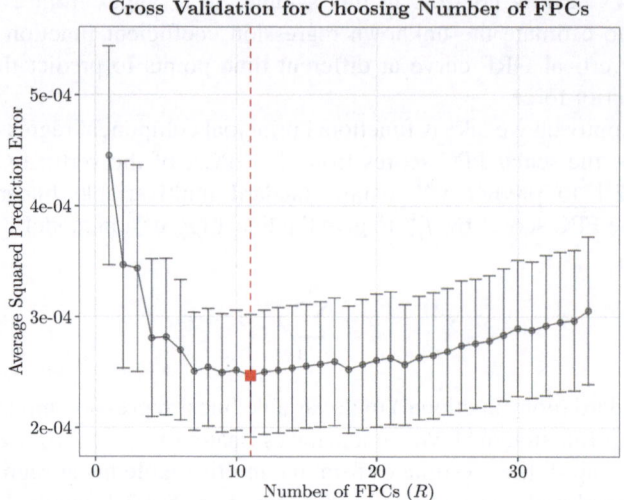

Fig. 5.8 The results of leave-one-out cross-validation to choose the number of FPCs to use in FPCR to predict the maximum anterior-posterior force

`fRegress.CV()` function and looping through a grid of values for λ, varying on a log scale. We find the optimum value to be $\log_{10}(\lambda) = 2.1$. The `pfr()` function uses a similar basis representation, but fitting is done in the generalised additive mixed model framework using the **mgcv** package [43]. For consistency, we also use 35 cubic B-spline basis functions with an integrated squared second derivative penalty. In `pfr()`, the model is fitted using restricted maximum likelihood (REML), so the smoothing parameter is chosen "automatically" (no manual loops are necessary). Figure 5.9c displays the final estimates from the FPCR, `fRegress()` and `pfr()` approaches, with associated 95% pointwise confidence intervals.

The three estimates of $\beta(t)$ in Fig. 5.9 generally represent an effect that is similar in magnitude and direction along the whole domain. However, the `pfr()` and `fRegress()` estimates are very similar (almost identical up to changes near the boundary of the domain), whereas the FPCR estimate exhibits more severe wiggles early and late in the movement. This is likely because the FPCs are a less flexible basis than the rich spline basis, and the means of regularisation is more crude (choosing a discrete truncation R vs a search for λ on a finer grid). We also note that the confidence intervals from `pfr()` are wider than those from `fRegress()`. This may be because the **mgcv** package uses Bayesian confidence intervals that account for both variance and (squared) bias, whereas the intervals in `fRegress()` neglect bias. To the best of our knowledge, the methods we have used to construct intervals for each approach neglect uncertainty in the hyperparameter selection for regularisation (i.e., we do not account for uncertainty due to selecting the number of FPCs for FPCR or the smoothing parameter in `fRegress()` and `pfr()`).

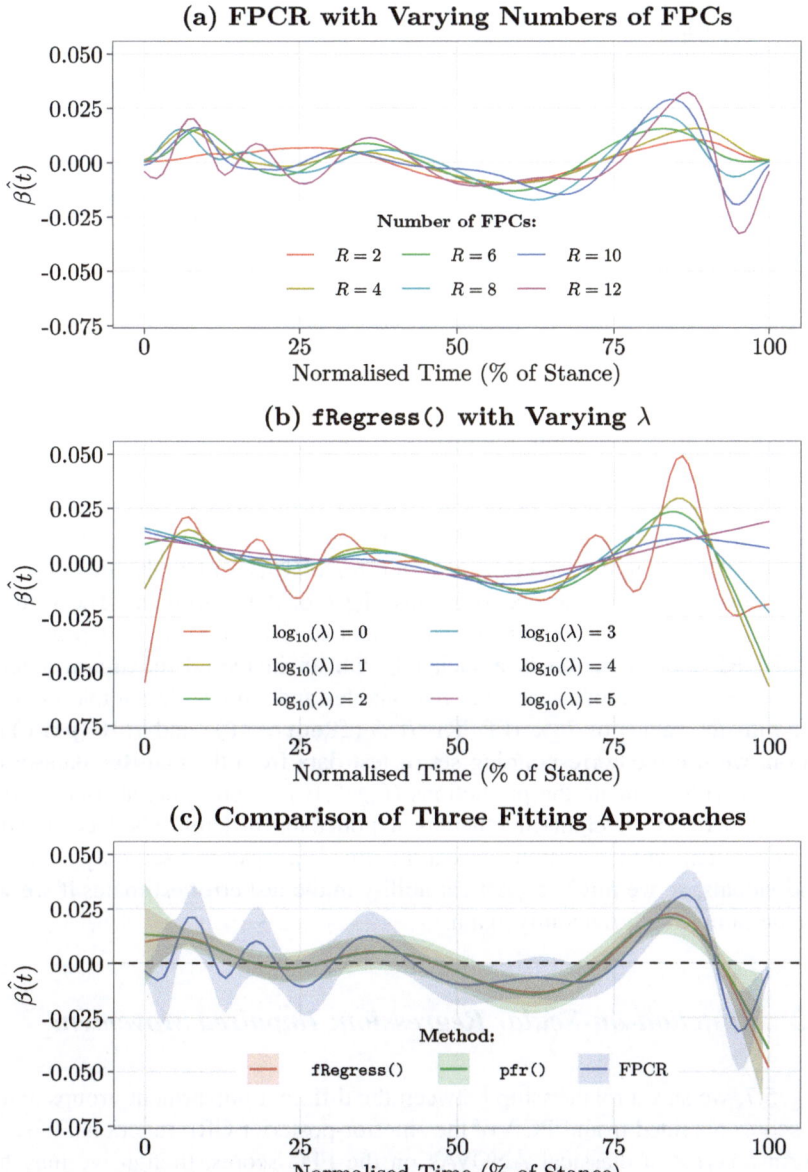

Fig. 5.9 (a) The estimated regression coefficient function $\widehat{\beta}(t)$ from the FPCR procedure using different numbers of FPCs. (b) The estimated regression coefficient function $\widehat{\beta}(t)$ from fRegress() using a number of different values for the smoothing parameter λ. (c) The best fits obtained from the three approaches: fRegress(), pfr() and FPCR. The solid lines represent the point estimates and the ribbons represent the 95% pointwise confidence intervals. For fRegress(), the smoothing parameter value $\log_{10}(\lambda) = 2.1$ is chosen by LOO-CV. Likewise, for FPCR, the optimum number of FPCs $R = 11$ is chosen by LOO-CV. For pfr(), the level of smoothing is chosen automatically via REML

Fig. 5.10 The absolute errors
of the test set predictions
using the three
scalar-on-function regression
models

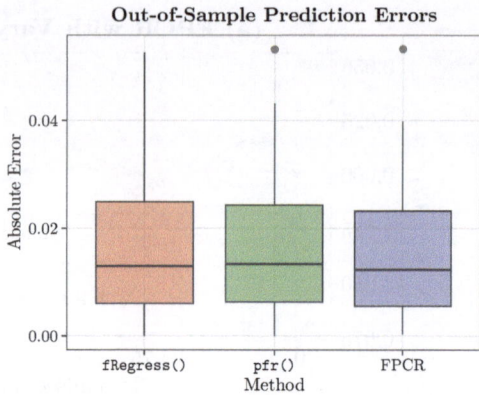

In terms of the application, the results of this scalar-on-function regression are
to be expected. In Fig. 5.9c, for all three estimates, the most prominent feature
in the estimated regression coefficient function is the peak between 75–100% of
the movement, indicating that this region in the vertical GRF curve is useful for
predicting the maximum anterior-posterior force. Unsurprisingly, the maximum
anterior-posterior force also occurs in this phase of the movement. The values of
$\beta(t)$ are positive in this region, meaning that an increased second peak in the
vertical GRF in this region is associated with an increased maximum anterior-
posterior force. The models provide reasonable (and similar) in-sample goodness
of fit, with R^2 values of 78% (FPCR), 78% (fRegress()) and 76% (pfr()). In
addition, we use the corresponding set of test data from the GaitRec dataset (see
TRAIN in [5]) to evaluate the predictions (Fig. 5.10). Overall, the absolute error is
small ($\approx$ 1% of body weight) and there is no noticeable difference between the three
approaches. This comes with the caveat that this is a small test set, only containing
64 individuals, so we might expect variability in the test error estimates if we were
to do the sample split randomly again.

5.4.2 Function-on-Scalar Regression: Impaired Movement

In Fig. 5.7, we saw a relationship between the different impairment groups and the
FPC scores obtained from FPCA of the anterior-posterior GRF functions. We could
perform a series of classical ANOVAs on the FPC scores, though we may have
problems summarising the results of multiple tests or correcting for Type-I errors.
Instead, we can formalise the comparison of the anterior-posterior GRF functions
between the groups by formulating a function-on-scalar regression with the same
form as in Chap. 4:

$$y_i(t) = \beta_0(t) + \sum_{p=1}^{5} x_{ip}\beta_p(t) + \epsilon_i(t),$$

where:

- $y_i(t)$ is the anterior-posterior force function for the ith individual,
- $\beta_0(t)$ is the intercept function,
- $x_{i1}, \ldots, x_{i5}$ are dummy-coded scalar covariates that represent membership of the healthy control and ankle, knee, hip and calcaneus impairment groups,
- $\beta_1(t), \ldots, \beta_5(t)$ are the corresponding regression coefficient functions for scalar covariates $x_{i1}, \ldots, x_{i5}$. We enforce the constraint $\sum_{p=1}^{5} \beta_p(t) = 0$ for all t, so that $\beta_p(t)$ represents the deviation of the pth group from the overall mean function, and
- $\epsilon_i(t)$ is the smooth functional random error term.

This is a one-way functional ANOVA model because we only have scalar covariates that represent different levels of the same factor variable. However, viewing it as a function-on-scalar regression model is a more general framework and would allow, e.g., a linear functional effect of walking speed to be included if we wanted to adjust for this variable in our comparison between the groups. We fit this model using four of the approaches described in Chap. 4:

1. **Two-Step Pointwise Estimation** [136, 137]: We simply fit a series of linear regression models using lm() at $t = 0, 1, \ldots, 100$ and then interpolate the pointwise estimates to produce the regression coefficient function estimates.[5]
2. **Penalised Ordinary Least Squares (P-OLS)** [4, 138]: This least-squares approach, where both the functional response and the regression coefficient functions are represented by basis expansions, is implemented in the fRegress() function in the **fda** package [118]. We use the same basis of 35 cubic B-splines to represent the regression coefficient functions, and choose a common smoothing parameter for them using cross-validation.
3. **Penalised Generalised Least Squares (P-GLS)** [138]: This approach is implemented in the fosr() function in the **refund** package [42]. The same basis of 35 cubic B-splines used to represent the data is chosen to represent the regression coefficient functions, but a separate smoothing parameter is chosen for each regression coefficient function.
4. **Functional Additive Mixed Model (FAMM)** [54, 135, 139]: This approach is implemented in the pffr() function in the **refund** package [42]. We use 35 cubic B-splines with a P-spline penalty [66] to represent the regression coefficient functions. Due to computational constraints, we do not model the error term as a smooth residual function. Hence, we implicitly assume that the errors are white noise rather than functions—this assumption should suffice for obtaining point estimates (and for the purpose of this case study, showcasing how these can be obtained), but will lead to poor uncertainty estimates because the error structure is incorrectly specified (see discussion in Greven and Scheipl [141] and Kokoszka and Reimherr [173]).

---

[5] We apply this approach manually using a for loop and the lm() function and also using fosr2s() from the **refund** package [42].

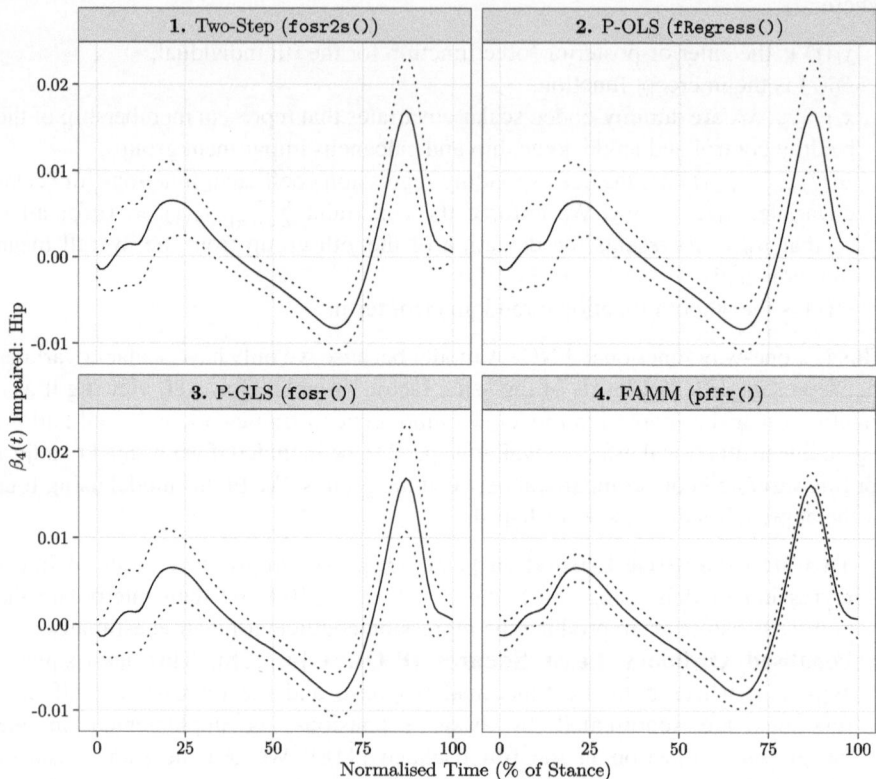

Fig. 5.11 Point estimates (solid lines) and 95% pointwise confidence intervals (dotted lines) for the regression coefficient function $\beta_4(t)$, which represents the deviation of the hip impairment group from the overall mean. The models are fitted using the four approaches described: (**1.**) Two-Step Pointwise Estimation (Two-Step) [136, 137], (**2.**) Penalised Ordinary Least Squares (P-OLS) [4, 138], (**3.**) Penalised Generalised Least Squares (P-GLS) [138], and (**4.**) Functional Additive Mixed Model (FAMM) [54, 135, 139]

The point estimates from all four approaches turn out to be very similar. Figure 5.11 displays the point estimates and approximate 95% pointwise confidence intervals for $\beta_4(t)$. As expected, the confidence intervals for the FAMM approach are too narrow because we have ignored residual auto-correlation across t. To obtain better uncertainty estimates with this approach, we could perform a bootstrap (see [54]).

To build simultaneous confidence bands shown in Fig. 5.12, we use an approach that was first proposed by Faraway [137] and Ruppert et al. [71] and is commonly employed in functional regression (e.g., see Degras [63], Crainiceanu et al. [174],

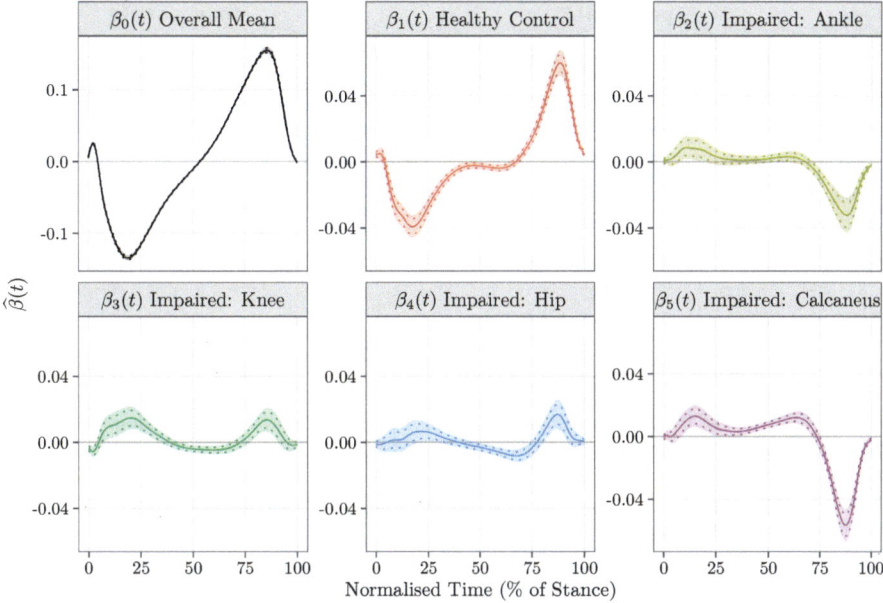

Fig. 5.12 Regression coefficient function estimates (solid lines), pointwise confidence intervals (dotted lines) and simultaneous confidence bands (shaded ribbons) obtained using a nonparametric bootstrapping and simulation approach [63, 71, 174–176]. The model fits are performed using the P-GLS method [138] with the `fosr()` function in the **refund** package

Park et al. [175], Cui et al. [176]). That is, for each p, we use a bootstrap and simulation to empirically approximate the distribution[6]

$$\max_{t \in [0,100]} \frac{|\widehat{\beta}_p(t) - \beta_p(t)|}{\widehat{\mathrm{SE}}\left(\widehat{\beta}_p(t)\right)},$$

and then construct confidence intervals

$$\widehat{\beta}_p(t) \pm \widehat{q}_{p,0.95}\widehat{\mathrm{SE}}\left(\widehat{\beta}_p(t)\right),$$

where $\widehat{q}_{p,0.95}$ is the 95th percentile of the empirical distribution. The simultaneous bands are shown as shaded ribbons in Fig. 5.12 and they are approximately 1.5 times as wide as the pointwise intervals (dotted lines)—we can view this as a "multiple comparisons correction" that provides coverage for the entire curve [63, 174]. The bands exclude 0 at several points, indicating statistical significance of each group's deviation from the overall mean. The magnitude and shape of $\widehat{\beta}_1(t)$ indicates

---

[6] This is the maximum of the classical Student's t-statistic for a regression coefficient $\beta_p(t)$ calculated pointwise at each $t \in [0, 100]$.

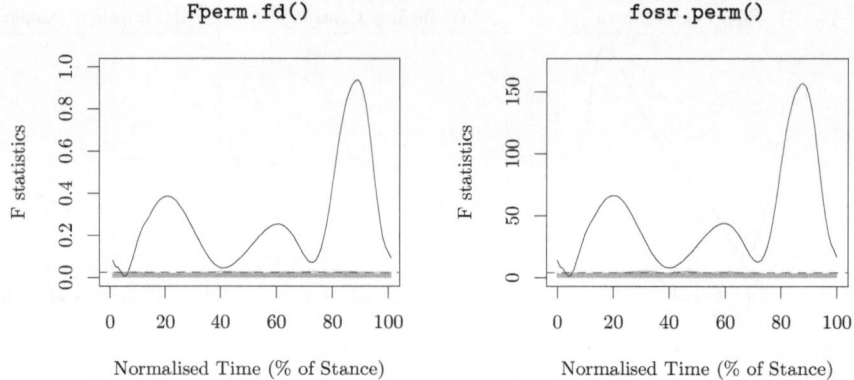

Fig. 5.13 Results of the F_{max} permutation test for the function-on-scalar regression model using the Fperm.fd() (left) and fosr.perm() (right) functions. The solid blue line represents the observed F-statistic function. The dashed red line indicates the critical value for the F_{max} test at the 5% level. The grey lines show F-statistic functions calculated on each permutation. In both cases, 400 permutations are used

a strong, statistically significant deviation of the healthy control group from the overall mean. This effect is most prominent around the instances of maximum braking and propulsive forces (approximately $t \in [12.5, 25\%]$ and $t \in [75, 87.5\%]$, respectively) and reflects the qualitative description provided by examining FPC1 and the FPC1 scores.

To jointly conclude about the overall effect of orthopaedic impairment, we use an F_{max} permutation test as described in Chap. 4 [20, 138]. The F_{max} test for the P-OLS and P-GLS methods is implemented in the Fperm.fd() and fosr.perm() functions in the **fda** and **refund** packages, respectively. Figure 5.13 displays the results of performing the test with both implementations. The results of both tests (ignoring different scaling) are almost identical—the observed F-statistic (solid blue line) exceeds the critical value for the F_{max} test (dashed red line) at almost every point in the domain, indicating a strong statistically significant relationship between orthopaedic impairment and the anterior-posterior GRF curves at almost every point in the stance phase.

5.5   Summary and Conclusions

This case study demonstrates that the conventional approach of performing FPCA and using the resulting scalar FPC scores in standard multivariable or multivariate statistical models often serves an applied researcher well and can be a very useful first step, especially when the data are smooth and can be well described by a small number of FPCs. However, there are more refined techniques within the FDA toolkit that can formalise relationships more concretely, providing increased statistical performance or enhanced interpretability. For example, in the case of impaired movement, FPCA assisted in describing differences in braking and propulsive force generation between the healthy controls and impaired conditions, which were modelled, quantified and interpreted more comprehensively using function-on-scalar regression. We also recommend trialling multiple approaches and software implementations, to visualise and compare their results as a sensitivity check and to understand the extent to which they agree. Some specific limitations of the case study are provided in Sect. 5.6.

5.6 Limitations

In addition to the limitations presented in Sect. 5.1.2, we note that:

- Individual uncertainty estimates presented in this section may have their own limitations, e.g., we have only provided pointwise confidence intervals in Sect. 5.4.1, some confidence intervals ignore bias in smoothed estimates and others neglect uncertainty due to smoothing/ hyperparameter selection.
- Although predicting the maximum anterior-posterior GRF from the vertical GRF presents as a tractable case for demonstrating scalar-on-function regression, we do not claim it to be an interesting scientific result or a useful endeavour.
- We have shown reasonable agreement between a variety of different approaches and implementations. However, we should acknowledge that our data present "favourable conditions" for applying FDA—they are smooth, sampled on a moderately dense grid without any missingness, and both subsets analysed comprise a reasonable number of subjects. We might not expect such agreement between different approaches under other, less favourable conditions.
- While we have presented functional regression models as natural progressions from exploratory applications of FPCA to highlight links between the techniques and aid understanding, we must note the dangers of "double dipping", i.e., forming hypotheses to test directly from an exploratory analysis of a set of data, and then testing these hypotheses on the same data.
- We have not considered any *function-on-function* regression models, but these could be used to model various relationships in the GaitRec data.
- We have focused on frequentist statistical approaches to functional regression, but Bayesian FDA approaches may provide an interesting alternative (see Crainiceanu and Goldsmith [23], Morris and Carroll [81], Morris [127], Goldsmith and Kitago [177]).
- We have employed off-the-shelf implementations from the widely-used **fda** and **refund** R packages, but that is not to say that other comparable implementations do not exist (e.g., using other R packages or other programming languages such as Python or MATLAB).

Despite these limitations we hope that this chapter has helped to showcase various practicalities of the methods and applications reviewed in Chaps. 2–4.

Bibliographic Notes

- Section 5.1.1 is a short and non-technical summary of the GaitRec data descriptor [5].
- The R code to perform the analysis was aided by examples in the monograph by Ramsay et al. [20]:
  - Code for fitting scalar-on-function models using fRegress() is provided on pp. 132–141.
  - A description of the calculation of confidence intervals for FPCR is contained on p. 143.
  - Fitting function-on-scalar models using fRegress() is detailed on pp. 147–149 and corresponding details on pointwise confidence intervals provided on pp. 157–158.
  - Details on the F_{max} permutation test and using the Fperm.fd() function are contained on p. 145 and pp. 168–169.
- The **refund** R package reference manual[7] contains full details for fitting models using the package.

---

[7] https://cran.r-project.org/web/packages/refund/refund.pdf.

Chapter 6
Future Directions of FDA in Biomechanics

Abstract This chapter gives a snapshot of sub-fields of FDA that are well-suited to analysing modern biomechanical data. Functional mixed-effects models allow the complex grouping and dependence structures (e.g., induced by multiple subjects being measured for repeated trials/sessions) that arise in large biomechanical datasets to be modelled appropriately. Multivariate FDA techniques provide advantages in analysing human movement data over their univariate counterparts, as they can capture co-variation between multiple joints. Finally, FDA provides direct access to examining the relationships between derivatives of functions and this is another interesting area to explore.

Keywords Functional mixed effects models · Multivariate functional data analysis · Differential equations · Dynamical systems

6.1 Functional Mixed Effects Models

The functional regression examples in Chap. 4 assumed independent functional data (i.e., through an implicit assumption that the smooth random error functions are independent), which, in modern applications, is unlikely to hold. Instead, dependence arises from grouping structures in the data, due to individuals being measured a number of times (e.g., performing a number of trials), being measured on both sides of the body, or even belonging to a cluster (e.g., a team or a school). These grouping structures induce correlations between curves that should be accounted for to achieve efficient estimation and to make correct inferences. For example, in the function-on-scalar regression model of vertical ground reaction force (vGRF) in Chap. 4, we modelled the average of a subject's trials on the left leg from a single standardised session, to align with the independence assumption [5]. However, we might wish to model every trial from multiple sessions bilaterally, without averaging or violating model assumptions. We may wish to quantify the variability between trials, sessions and sides of the body, while making correct inferences about the effect of orthopaedic impairment, or conditions that change between sessions.

© The Author(s), under exclusive license to Springer Nature Switzerland AG 2024   73
E. Gunning et al., *Functional Data Analysis in Biomechanics*,
SpringerBriefs in Statistics, https://doi.org/10.1007/978-3-031-68862-1_6

For scalar outcomes, linear mixed effects models (LMMs) offer a common and convenient way to account for such grouping structures, using the notion of fixed and random effects [75]. Faraway [178, p. 195] defines a fixed effect as "an unknown constant that we try to estimate from the data". In contrast, a random effect can better be understood as a random parameter that is a draw (or realisation) from a larger population distribution, such that it makes more sense to estimate parameters that describe this distribution rather than estimate the individual random effects' values [178, p. 195]. Although this distinction is imperfect, and fixed and random effects are used in several ways nowadays [179, Chap. 13], it is useful for contextualising the potential utility of LMMs in biomechanics and human movement research. For example, it might be appropriate to treat an individual athlete as randomly drawn from a wider population of athletes (in other words, if we re-collected our sample, it may contain different athletes), whose characteristics we would like to estimate. Instead of estimating a fixed effect for each specific athlete, we might be concerned with characterising, more generally, how an outcome (or the effect of a covariate on it) varies randomly from athlete to athlete.

The functional analogue of LMMs, *functional* linear mixed effects models (FLMMs) are popular within FDA, and a number of approaches have been proposed [127, 135] (for reviews, see Liu and Guo [49] and Morris [22, Sect. 5.5]). An elementary example is to extend the function-on-scalar regression model to a repeated-measures setting, by including a functional random intercept. If individuals were measured multiple times (e.g., for repeated trials), the functional random intercept accounts for each individual having a different average (function). Let $y_{ij}(t)$ represent the jth observed function from the ith individual, $i = 1, ..., N$ and $j = 1, ..., J$, and x_{ijp} the associated scalar covariates $p = 1, ..., P$. The model becomes

$$y_{ij}(t) = \beta_0(t) + \sum_{p=1}^{P} x_{ijp}\beta_p(t) + u_i(t) + \epsilon_{ij}(t), \tag{6.1.1}$$

where the regression coefficient functions $\beta_0(t), ..., \beta_P(t)$ are as before, and are now called the "fixed functional effects" in the model; $u_i(t)$ is the functional random intercept for subject i and $\epsilon_{ij}(t)$ is the curve-specific random error function. The $u_i(t)$ term is treated as a smooth stochastic process, similar to the $\epsilon_{ij}(t)$, and it accounts for correlation between different curves from the same subject. Put simply, by adding a different mean for each subject into the model, we can then conceivably view the deviations of repeated trials around this mean (i.e., the residual errors $\epsilon_{ij}(t)$) as independent, thus satisfying modelling assumptions. More complex functional random effects structures are possible e.g., that account for multiple nested layers of variability [15, 35, 133], or curves for each individual that have a distinct ordering in time [15, 96, 180]. Although detailing specific approaches to fitting FLMMs is beyond the scope of this book, generally they rely on basis function representations of the parameters and formulating of the model that are based on scalar LMMs for estimation and inference [22, 49, 127, 139, 141].

Quantifying various sources and levels of randomness, e.g., being able to simultaneously handle trial-to-trial and athlete-to-athlete variability, can inform skill, coordination and injury rehabilitation research,. However, FLMMs have received surprisingly little attention in applied biomechanics settings. Different methodological work on inference for functional data in repeated measures/ mixed-effects settings have been motivated by or demonstrated on orthoses datasets [33, 181, 182]. Goldsmith and Kitago [177] used a FLMM to model biomechanical data on upper extremity motor control in stroke patients, where kinematic data of hand position during a reaching motion to eight separate targets were recorded. They estimated the effects of motor impairment and the target number on the reaching trajectories, while accounting for fixed covariates such as side (dominant vs. non-dominant) and subject-level functional random effects jointly in a Bayesian framework. More recently, Volkmann et al. [183] showed an example of multivariate FLMMs applied to sports science data from snooker, where the effect of a training programme on movement trajectories of snooker players was investigated (a fixed effect), while accounting for variation between players, between sessions and between shots using functional random effects. A possible reason for the limited use of FLMMs in applied biomechanics and human movement research is that they are statistically advanced and may be deemed unnecessarily complex for some applications, e.g., when compared with averaging curves and applying techniques for independent functional data; they can also be computationally expensive to fit [49, 133, 177]. However, they may be used more widely in the future as their flexibility for handling the complexities of modern biomechanical data is recognised.

6.2   Multivariate Functional Data

So far, we have generally outlined techniques for analysing univariate functional data (i.e., single functional variables). However, some examples lend themselves more naturally to being treated as *multivariate* (or *vector-valued*) *functional data*. For example, it often makes sense to simultaneously analyse a pair or triple of joint angles observed concurrently during a movement (e.g., knee and hip angles), and to treat two-dimensional [177, 183] or three-dimensional [105, 184] position coordinates collectively as a single object. We typically refer to multivariate functional data as comprising multiple *dimensions*, where each dimension is a different functional variable. Figure 6.1 displays some examples of multivariate functional data arising in biomechanics. Rather than take the standard approach of plotting the functional data from each dimension against time, the dimensions are plotted against one another to reveal patterns and relationships between them. When the functions in each dimension represent the angle of a different joint, this visualisation is known as an *angle-angle* diagram, and can be used to assess inter-joint coordination in biomechanics (see Lamb and Bartlett [185, Sect. 2]). The concept of multivariate functional data analysis is useful beyond the analysis of joint angles too. For example, "movement signatures" in sports can also be realised by multiple technical

(a) Juggling

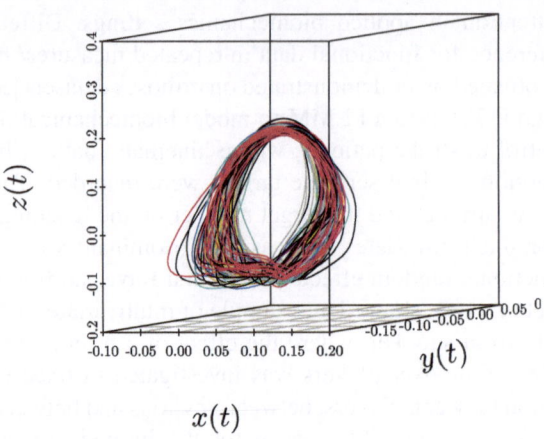

(b) Children's Gait   **(c) Running**

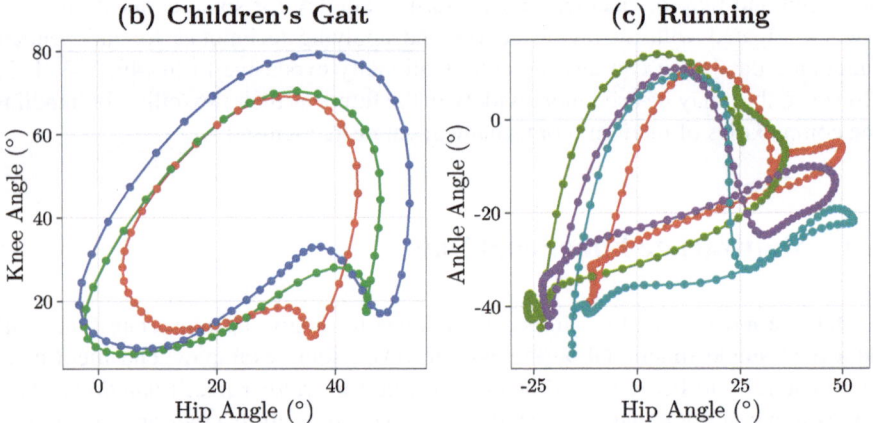

Fig. 6.1 Three examples of multivariate functional data arising in biomechanics. In each case, the dimensions of the multivariate functional data are plotted against one another, rather than against time. (**a**): The three-dimensional co-ordinates of the juggler's index finger in the juggling dataset [8, 103]. (**b**): Hip and knee angles from the children's gait dataset [2–4, 6]. (**c**): Hip and ankle angles from a study of coordination in running by Trounson et al. [187]

variables, such as an object's trajectory or the force applied to it. These technical variables can be heterogeneous (e.g., comprise kinetics and kinematics) and can represent cues for skill, technique or coordination. Warmenhoven et al. [186] demonstrated this idea in rowing, treating the rower's force curve and the horizontal angle of the oar jointly as a bivariate functional data object, providing a natural representation of the rower's "force-angle profile".

Applications to biomechanics have primarily used FPCA for bivariate functional data, *bivariate FPCA* (BFPCA), which takes the cross-covariance between the dimensions of the bivariate function into account and thus can extract components of variation that are common across the two dimensions. BFPCA has been used to analyse couples of joints (and hence, coordination) [187, 188], knee angle and knee moment jointly [189], and pairs of technical variables in rowing [186] and weightlifting [190]. Functional regression models can also be multivariate (this was the case in the applications by Goldsmith and Kitago [177] and Volkmann et al. [183]), and functional canonical correlation analysis (FCCA) is a technique for bivariate functional data that has been used to reveal the ways in which pairs of functions, such as hip and knee angles, are correlated [3, 4].

From a methodological perspective, Wang et al. [62] and Koner and Staicu [191] class multivariate functional data as *next-generation functional data*, because they have become increasingly popular (many fields now collect multiple data streams in parallel) and they pose novel challenges and opportunities for research. For example, methodology has been developed to allow FPCA to be applied to multivariate functional data where the dimensions are measured in different units (e.g., joint angles and joint moments) [36] and observed on different domains (e.g., images and curves) [38]. We expect further developments to arise from applications in biomechanics and human movement research, where several streams of functional data are routinely collected in parallel, often by different recording technologies (e.g., force plates, motion capture systems and sensors).

6.3 Dynamics and Functional Data

The final direction that we will mention is *dynamics* in FDA. The possibility of using derivatives in FDA stems directly from its key characterising idea—by viewing each set of measurements as arising from a smooth underlying function, we naturally have access to the rates of change of that function. In this context, we will refer to *dynamic modelling* as the process of using FDA tools to directly study the relationship between a function and a number of its derivatives to understand its temporal evolution [4, 20, 47]. In applied mathematics, models of this type are known as *differential equations* and, more generally, when they comprise multiple equations they are known as *dynamical systems*. Ramsay [192] first proposed to combine the observations of a function and its derivatives with the functional regression tools described in Chap. 4, to estimate an underlying differential equation. This approach was called Principal Differential Analysis (PDA) [192]. As noted by Ramsay [192], finding a differential equation that fits a set of functional data well has two main practical advantages—its solutions can be used as basis functions to represent the data, and its parameters can be used to understand the underlying dynamics. In subsequent publications, PDA was used in human movement applications to study the biomechanics of speaking [20], handwriting [20, 47, 193] and juggling [194].

Fig. 6.2 A three-dimensional phase-plane plot of the juggling data. Here we have taken the z coordinate from a single trial, denoted by $z(t)$. We have then plotted it against its first and second temporal derivatives, denoted by $Dz(t)$ and $D^2z(t)$, respectively

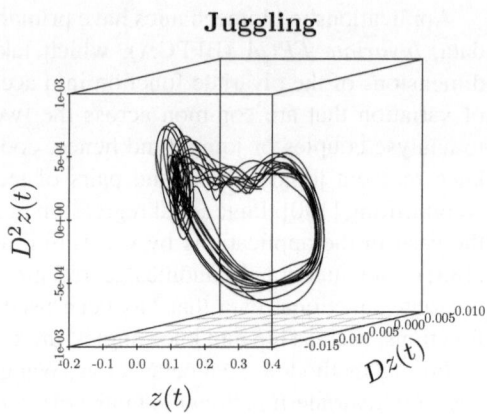

Dynamic FDA models have not yet received attention in applied biomechanics fields (e.g., sports, clinical biomechanics and rehabilitation) in the way other techniques, such as FPCA, have. This is despite theories and tools used in coordination research (e.g., [129, 195]) also being based on dynamical systems ideas. While a full example of dynamic modelling is beyond the scope of this chapter, we present the *phase-plane plot* (or *portrait*), which is the graphical technique of plotting a function against its derivative or one of its derivatives against another (Fig. 6.2). Here we have taken the z coordinate of the juggler's index finger for a single trial, consisting of 12 cycles. We have then calculated its first and second derivatives with respect to time, denoting them by $Dz(t)$ and $D^2z(t)$, respectively. Each cycle forms an approximately-circular orbit in the phase-plane, but the relationship among the derivatives appears intrinsically complex as there are cusps and curves in the phase-plane representation. To decipher the underlying relationship more formally, the PDA approach would involve estimating a functional regression model that describes $D^2z(t)$ as a function of $z(t)$ and $Dz(t)$. For an application of phase-plane plotting on the children's gait dataset, see Ramsay et al. [20, p. 160, Fig. 10.6].

Interestingly, phase-plane plots were identified as a visualisation tool for joint kinematics in human locomotion over 25 years ago [196]. In addition, *continuous relative phase (CRP)*, a prevalent technique used to study coordination with application in rehabilitation, injury prevention and sports performance analysis, is based on analysis of joint angles or segments in the phase-plane [195]. Clearly, there is substantial interest in understanding biomechanical data from the perspective of dynamical systems, and it remains to be seen what impact the tools of FDA can have.

6.4 Conclusion

In this text, we have reviewed the core techniques and applications of FDA in biomechanics and human movement research to date. With recent increases in the volume, variety and complexity of biomechanical data, FDA provides an important set of tools for researchers to learn about movement. As demonstrated in all of our examples, FDA preserves the time-dependent structure of continuous biomechanical data, which sets it apart from many contemporary machine learning approaches. Some of the techniques we have described, such as FPCA and functional regression, are generalisations of familiar statistical techniques to the functional setting, tailored to allow properties such as smoothness to be imposed. Others, such as registration, do not have a multivariate analogue, and specifically address challenges posed by functional data. With these combined, FDA provides a toolkit for processing, exploration, prediction and inference with continuous biomechanical data.

The techniques we have described aim to capture the majority of the applications of FDA to biomechanics to date. Therefore, we have given an introductory overview of each technique and provided examples on real biomechanical datasets, rather than simply list specific applications. We have made a connection to extensions of these techniques—many of which have been motivated by data in adjacent biomedical fields—as they hold significant promise for progressing biomechanics as an area of application. It must be noted that there are other topics in FDA that could have been given more focus; brief discussions of clustering and classification arose within the context of FPCA and functional regression, however these are important areas of FDA research themselves. The future directions in this final chapter give a short overview of sub-fields of FDA that may have an impact on future biomechanics and human movement research. We acknowledge that there are other valuable use-cases that we might have failed to mention (e.g., test-retest and reliability methods using FDA [197], and directional FDA approaches that explicitly account for the circular nature of joint angles [198, 199]), and that others will emerge, driven by real-world problems in biomechanics.

To conclude, human movement biomechanics was one of the earliest areas of practical application for FDA methods and today it remains a growing area, with many exciting research opportunities. We hope that this review will act as catalyst to further accelerate its growth.

References

1. J.O. Ramsay, When the data are functions. Psychometrika **47**(4), 379–396 (1982)
2. J.A. Rice, B.W. Silverman, Estimating the mean and covariance structure nonparametrically when the data are curves. J. R. Stat. Soc. B Met. **53**(1), 233–243 (1991)
3. S.E. Leurgans, R.A. Moyeed, B.W. Silverman, Canonical correlation analysis when the data are curves. J. R. Stat. Soc. B Met. **55**(3), 725–740 (1993)
4. J.O. Ramsay, B.W. Silverman, *Functional Data Analysis*. Springer Series in Statistics, 2nd edn. (Springer-Verlag, Berlin, 2005)
5. B. Horsak, D. Slijepcevic, A. Raberger, C. Schwab, M. Worisch, M. Zeppelzauer, GaitRec, a large-scale ground reaction force dataset of healthy and impaired gait. Sci. Data **7**(1), 143 (2020)
6. R.A. Olshen, E.N. Biden, M.P. Wyatt, D.H. Sutherland, Gait analysis and the bootstrap. Ann. Stat. **17**(4), 1419–1440 (1989)
7. J.S. Marron, J.O. Ramsay, L.M. Sangalli, A.Srivastava, Statistics of time warpings and phase variations. Electron. J. Stat. **8**(2), 1697–1702 (2014)
8. J.O. Ramsay, P. Gribble, S. Kurtek, Description and processing of functional data arising from juggling trajectories. Electron. J. Stat. **8**(2), 1811–1816 (2014)
9. D.A. Winter, *Biomechanics of Human Movement* (Wiley, New York, 1979)
10. A. Phinyomark, G. Petri, E. Ibáñez-Marcelo***, S.T. Osis, R. Ferber, Analysis of big data in gait biomechanics: Current trends and future directions. J. Med. Biol. Eng. **38**(2), 244–260 (2018)
11. R. Ferber, S.T. Osis, J.L. Hicks, S.L. Delp, Gait biomechanics in the era of data science. J. Biomech. **49**(16), 3759–3761 (2016)
12. C. Richter, M. O'Reilly, E. Delahunt, Machine learning in sports science: challenges and opportunities. Sports Biomech. **0**(0), 1–7 (2021)
13. F. Horst, D. Slijepcevic, M. Simak, W.I. Schöllhorn, Gutenberg Gait Database, a ground reaction force database of level overground walking in healthy individuals. Sci. Data **8**(1), 232 (2021)
14. E. Halilaj, A. Rajagopal, M. Fiterau, J.L. Hicks, T.J. Hastie, S.L. Delp, Machine learning in human movement biomechanics: Best practices, common pitfalls, and new opportunities. J. Biomech. **81**, 1–11 (2018)
15. J. Lee, G. Li, W.F. Christensen, G. Collins, M. Seeley, A.E. Bowden, D.T. Fullwood, J. Goldsmith, Functional data analyses of gait data measured using in-shoe sensors. Stat. Biosci. **11**(2), 288–313 (2019)

© The Author(s), under exclusive license to Springer Nature Switzerland AG 2024
E. Gunning et al., *Functional Data Analysis in Biomechanics*,
SpringerBriefs in Statistics, https://doi.org/10.1007/978-3-031-68862-1

16. K. Hébert-Losier, A. Pini, S. Vantini, J.Strandberg, K. Abramowicz, L. Schelin, C.K. Häger, One-leg hop kinematics 20 years following anterior cruciate ligament rupture: data revisited using functional data analysis. Clin. Biomech. **30**(10), 1153–1161 (2015)

17. J. Warmenhoven, N. Bargary, D. Liebl, A.J. Harrison, M.A. Robinson, E. Gunning, G. Hooker, PCA of waveforms and functional PCA: a primer for biomechanics. J. Biomech. **116**, 110106 (2021)

18. P. Besse, J.O. Ramsay, Principal components analysis of sampled functions. Psychometrika **51**(2), 285–311 (2016)

19. D.B. Clarkson, C. Fraley, C. Gu, J.O. Ramsay, *S+Functional Data Analysis: User's Manual for Windows* (Springer, Berlin, 2005)

20. J.O. Ramsay, G. Hooker, S. Graves, *Functional Data Analysis with R and MATLAB*. Use R! (Springer-Verlag, Berlin, 2009)

21. J.L. Wang, J.M. Chiou, H.G. Müller, Functional data analysis. Ann. Rev. Stat. Appl. **3**(1), 257–295 (2016)

22. J.S. Morris, Functional regression. Ann. Rev. Stat. Appl. **2**, 321–359 (2015)

23. C.M. Crainiceanu, J.A. Goldsmith, Bayesian functional data analysis using WinBUGS. J. Stat. Softw. **32**(1), 1–33 (2010)

24. N. Coffey, A.J. Harrison, O.A. Donoghue, K. Hayes, Common functional principal components analysis: A new approach to analyzing human movement data. Hum. Mov. Sci. **30**(6), 1144–1166 (2011)

25. B.W. Silverman, Some aspects of the spline smoothing approach to non-parametric regression curve fitting. J. R. Stat. Soc. B Met. **47**(1), 1–21 (1985)

26. I.T. Jolliffe, *Principal Component Analysis*. Springer Series in Statistics (Springer-Verlag, Berlin, 1986)

27. W. Ryan, A.J. Harrison, K. Hayes, Functional data analysis of knee joint kinematics in the vertical jump. Sports Biomech. **5**(1), 121–138 (2006)

28. P.P.Y. Wu, N. Sterkenburg, K. Everett, D.W. Chapman, N. White, K. Mengersen, Predicting fatigue using countermovement jump force-time signatures: PCA can distinguish neuromuscular versus metabolic fatigue. PLoS One **14**(7), e0219295 (2019)

29. J.L. McKay, T.D.J. Welch, B. Vidakovic, L.H. Ting, Statistically significant contrasts between EMG waveforms revealed using wavelet-based functional ANOVA. J. Neurophysiol. **109**, 591–602 (2012)

30. S. Ullah, C.F. Finch, Applications of functional data analysis: a systematic review. BMC Med. Res. Methodol. **13**(1), 43 (2013)

31. J. Dannenmaier, C. Kaltenbach, T.Kölle, G. Krischak, Application of functional data analysis to explore movements: walking, running and jumping - a systematic review. Gait Posture **77**, 182–189 (2020)

32. J. Warmenhoven, S. Cobley, C. Draper, A.J. Harrison, N. Bargary, R. Smith, Considerations for the use of functional principal components analysis in sports biomechanics: examples from on-water rowing. Sports Biomech. **18**(3), 317–341 (2019)

33. B. Zhang, R. Twycross-Lewis, H. Großmann, D. Morrissey, Testing gait with ankle-foot orthoses in children with cerebral palsy by using functional mixed-effects analysis of variance. Sci. Rep. **7**(1), 11081 (2017)

34. C.Z. Di, C.M. Crainiceanu, B.S. Caffo, N.M. Punjabi, Multilevel functional principal component analysis. Ann. Appl. Stat. **3**(1), 458–488 (2009)

35. H. Shou, V. Zipunnikov, C.M. Crainiceanu, S. Greven, Structured functional principal component analysis. Biometrics **71**(1), 247–257 (2015)

36. J. Jacques, C. Preda, Model-based clustering for multivariate functional data. Comput. Stat. Data Anal. **71**, 92–106 (2014)

37. J.M. Chiou, Y.T. Chen, Y.F. Yang, Multivariate functional principal component analysis: a normalization approach. Stat. Sinica **24**(4), 1571–1596 (2014)

38. C. Happ, S. Greven, Multivariate functional principal component analysis for data observed on different (dimensional) domains. J. Am. Stat. Assoc. **113**(522), 649–659 (2018)

39. L.M. Sangalli, P. Secchi, S. Vantini, V. Vitelli, k-mean alignment for curve clustering. Comput. Stat. Data Anal. **54**(5), 1219–1233 (2010)
40. A. Srivastava, W. Wu, S. Kurtek, E. Klassen, J.S. Marron, Registration of functional data using Fisher-Rao metric (2011). arXiv:1103.3817 [math, stat]
41. C.M. Crainiceanu, J. Goldsmith, A. Leroux, E. Cui, *Functional Data Analysis with R* (Chapman & Hall/CRC, London, 2024)
42. J. Goldsmith, F. Scheipl, L. Huang, J. Wrobel, C.Z. Di, J. Gellar, J. Harezlak, M.W. McLean, B. Swihart, L. Xiao, C.M. Crainiceanu, P.T. Reiss, Y. Chen, S. Greven, L. Huo, M.G. Kundu, S.Y. Park, D.L. Miller, A.M. Staicu, *refund: Regression with functional data* (2022). https://CRAN.R-project.org/package=refund. R package version 0.1-24
43. S.N. Wood, Fast stable restricted maximum likelihood and marginal likelihood estimation of semiparametric generalized linear models. J. R. Stat. Soc. B Met. **73**(1), 3–36 (2011)
44. J. Gertheiss, D.Rügamer, B.X.W. Liew, S. Greven, Functional data analysis: an introduction and recent developments (2023). *arXiv:2312.05523v1 [stat.ME]*
45. E.A. Crane, D. Childers, G. Gerstner, E. Rothman, Functional data analysis for biomechanics. Theor. Biomech. (2011)
46. A.J. Harrison, Applications of functional data analysis in sport biomechanics. ISBS - Conference Proceedings Archive (2014)
47. J.O. Ramsay, B.W. Silverman, *Applied Functional Data Analysis: Methods and Case Studies.* Springer Series in Statistics (Springer-Verlag, Berlin, 2002)
48. C.M. Crainiceanu, B. Caffo, J. Morris, Multilevel functional data analysis, in *The SAGE Handbook of Multilevel Modeling* (SAGE Publications Ltd, New York, 2013), pp. 223–248
49. Z. Liu, W. Guo, Functional mixed effects models. WIREs Comput. Stat. **4**(6), 527–534 (2012)
50. P.T. Reiss, R.T. Ogden, Functional principal component regression and functional partial least squares. J. Am. Stat. Assoc. **102**(479), 984–996 (2007)
51. H.L. Shang, A survey of functional principal component analysis. AStA Adv. Stat. Anal. **98**(2), 121–142 (2014)
52. H. Sørensen, J. Goldsmith, L.M. Sangalli, An introduction with medical applications to functional data analysis. Stat. Med. **32**(30), 5222–5240 (2013)
53. N. Coffey, J. Hinde, Analyzing time-course microarray data using functional data analysis - a review. Stat. Appl. Genet. Mol. Biol. (2011)
54. A. Bauer, F. Scheipl, H. Küchenhoff, A.A. Gabriel, An introduction to semiparametric function-on-scalar regression. Stat. Model. **18**(3–4), 346–364 (2018)
55. E. Gunning, *Statistical modelling of second-generation functional data with application in biomechanics and human movement research.* Ph.D. Thesis, University of Limerick, 2024
56. L.A. Prosser, S.C.K. Lee, M.F. Barbe, A.F. VanSant, R.T. Lauer, Trunk and hip muscle activity in early walkers with and without cerebral palsy – A frequency analysis. J. Electromyogr. Kinesiol. **20**(5), 851–859 (2010)
57. D. Liebl, S. Willwacher, J. Hamill, G.P. Brüggemann, Ankle plantarflexion strength in rearfoot and forefoot runners: a novel clusteranalytic approach. Hum. Mov. Sci. **35**, 104–120 (2014)
58. J. Warmenhoven, A.J. Harrison, M.A. Robinson, J. Vanrenterghem, N. Bargary, R. Smith, S. Cobley, C. Draper, C. Donnelly, T. Pataky, A force profile analysis comparison between functional data analysis, statistical parametric mapping and statistical non-parametric mapping in on-water single sculling. J. Sci. Med. Sport **21**(10), 1100–1105 (2018)
59. S. Kurtek, W. Wu, G.E. Christensen, A. Srivastava, Segmentation, alignment and statistical analysis of biosignals with application to disease classification. J. Appl. Stat. **40**(6), 1270–1288 (2013)
60. O.A. Donoghue, A.J. Harrison, N. Coffey, K. Hayes, Functional data analysis of running kinematics in chronic Achilles tendon injury. Med. Sci. Sports Exerc. **40**(7), 1323–1335 (2008)
61. J.O. Ramsay, C.J. Dalzell, Some tools for functional data analysis. J. R. Stat. Soc. B Met. **53**(3), 539–572 (1991)

62. J.L. Wang, J.M. Chiou, H.G. Mueller, Review of functional data analysis. Ann. Rev. Stat. Appl. **3**, 257–295 (2016)
63. D. Degras, Simultaneous confidence bands for the mean of functional data. WIREs Comput. Stat. **9**(3), e1397 (2017)
64. J. Røislien, Ø. Skare, M. Gustavsen, N.L. Broch, L. Rennie, A. Opheim, Simultaneous estimation of effects of gender, age and walking speed on kinematic gait data. Gait Posture **30**(4), 441–445 (2009)
65. M. Sangeux, E. Passmore, G. Gomez, J. Balakumar, H.K. Graham, Slipped capital femoral epiphysis, fixation by single screw in situ: a kinematic and radiographic study. Clin. Biomech. **29**(5), 523–530 (2014)
66. P.H.C. Eilers, B.D. Marx, Flexible smoothing with B-splines and penalties. Stat. Sci. **11**(2), 89–121, (1996)
67. K. Hébert-Losier, L. Schelin, E. Tengman, A. Strong, C.K. Häger, Curve analyses reveal altered knee, hip, and trunk kinematics during drop–jumps long after anterior cruciate ligament rupture. The Knee **25**(2), 226–239 (2018)
68. K. Abramowicz, C.K. Häger, A. Pini, L. Schelin, S.S. deLuna, S. Vantini, Nonparametric inference for functional-on-scalar linear models applied to knee kinematic hop data after injury of the anterior cruciate ligament. Scand. J. Stat. **45**(4), 1036–1061 (2018)
69. C. Baumgart, M.W. Hoppe, J. Freiwald, Phase-ppecific ground reaction force analyses of bilateral and unilateral jumps in patients with ACL reconstruction. Orthop. J. Sports Med. **5**(6) (2017)
70. F. O'Sullivan, A statistical perspective on ill-posed inverse problems. Stat. Sci. **1**(4), 502–518 (1986)
71. D. Ruppert, M.P. Wand, R.J. Carroll, *Semiparametric Regression*. Cambridge Series in Statistical and Probabilistic Mathematics (Cambridge University Press, Cambridge, 2003)
72. A. Page, G. Ayala, M.T. León, M.F. Peydro, J.M. Prat, Normalizing temporal patterns to analyze sit-to-stand movements by using registration of functional data. J. Biomech. **39**(13), 2526–2534 (2006)
73. P. Craven, G. Wahba, Smoothing noisy data with spline functions. Numer. Math. **31**(4), 377–403 (1978)
74. T. Hastie, R. Tibshirani, J. Friedman, *The Elements of Statistical Learning*, 2nd edn. (Springer, Berlin, 2009)
75. N.M. Laird, J.H. Ware, Random-effects models for longitudinal cata. Biometrics **38**(4), 963–974 (1982)
76. D. Bates, M.Mächler, B. Bolker, S. Walker, Fitting linear mixed-effects models using lme4. J. Stat. Softw. **67**(1), 1–48 (2015)
77. M.P. Wand, Smoothing and mixed models. Comput. Stat. **18**(2), 223–249 (2003)
78. L.N. Berry, N.E. Helwig, Cross-validation, information theory, or maximum likelihood? A comparison of tuning methods for penalized splines. Stats **4**(3), 701–724 (2021)
79. N. Coffey, *Functional principal components analysis in a linear mixed effects model framework*. Ph.D. Thesis, University of Limerick, 2008
80. K. Allison, S.E. Salomoni, K.L. Bennell, T.V. Wrigley, F. Hug, B. Vicenzino, A. Grimaldi, P.W. Hodges, Hip abductor muscle activity during walking in individuals with gluteal tendinopathy. Scand. J. Med. Sci. Sports **28**(2), 686–695 (2018)
81. J.S. Morris, R.J. Carroll, Wavelet-based functional mixed models. J. R. Stat. Soc. B Met. **68**(2), 179–199 (2006)
82. D. Pigoli, L.M. Sangalli, Wavelets in functional data analysis: Estimation of multidimensional curves and their derivatives. Comput. Stat. Data Anal. **56**(6), 1482–1498 (2012)
83. G.M. James, C.A. Sugar, Clustering for sparsely sampled functional data. J. Am. Stat. Assoc. **98**(462), 397–408 (2003)
84. F. Yao, H.G. Müller, J.L. Wang, Functional data analysis for sparse longitudinal data. J. Am. Stat. Assoc. **100**, 577–590 (2005)
85. T. Dos'Santos, P. Comfort, P.A. Jones, Average of trial peaks versus peak of average profile: impact on change of direction biomechanics. Sports Biomech. **19**, 483–492 (2020)

86. J. Wrobel, A. Bauer, E. McDonnell, J. Goldsmith, *registr: Curve registration for exponential family functional data* (2022). https://CRAN.R-project.org/package=registr, R package version 1.0.0

87. A. Kneip, J.O. Ramsay, Combining registration and fitting for functional models. J. Am. Stat. Assoc. **103**(483), 1155–1165 (2008)

88. A. Kneip, T. Gasser, Statistical tools to analyze data representing a sample of curves. Ann. Stat. **20**(3), 1266–1305 (1992)

89. T. Gasser, A. Kneip, Searching for structure in curve sample. J. Am. Stat. Assoc. **90**(432), 1179–1188 (1995)

90. M.A.M. Zin, A.S. Rambely, N.M. Ariff, Effectiveness of landmark and continuous registrations in reducing inter- and intrasubject phase variability. IEEE Access **8**, 216003–216017 (2020)

91. J.S. Marron, J.O. Ramsay, L.M. Sangalli, A. Srivastava, Functional data analysis of amplitude and phase variation. Stat. Sci. **30**(4), 468–484 (2015)

92. A. Srivastava, E. Klassen, S.H. Joshi, I.H. Jermyn, Shape analysis of elastic curves in Euclidean spaces. IEEE Trans. Pattern Anal. Mach. Intell. **33** (7), 1415–1428 (2011)

93. H. Wagner, A. Kneip, Nonparametric registration to low-dimensional function spaces. Comput. Stat. Data Anal. **138**, 49–63 (2019)

94. E.C. Honert, T.C. Pataky, Timing of gait events affects whole trajectory analyses: a statistical parametric mapping sensitivity analysis of lower limb biomechanics. J. Biomech. **119**, 110329 (2021)

95. D. Poss, H. Wagner, Analysis of juggling data: registering data to principal components to explain amplitude variation. Electron. J. Stat. **8**(2), 1825–1834 (2014)

96. J. Park, M.K. Seeley, D. Francom, C.S. Reese, J.T. Hopkins, Functional vs. traditional analysis in biomechanical gait data: an alternative statistical approach. J. Hum. Kinet. **60**, 39–49 (2017)

97. E.A. Crane, R.B. Cassidy, E.D. Rothman, G.E. Gerstner, Effect of registration on cyclical kinematic data. J. Biomech. **43**(12), 2444–2447 (2010)

98. H. Sadeghi, P. Allard, K. Shafie, P.A. Mathieu, S. Sadeghi, F. Prince, J.O. Ramsay, Reduction of gait data variability using curve registration. Gait Posture **12**(3), 257–264 (2000)

99. S. Moudy, C. Richter, S. Strike, Landmark registering waveform data improves the ability to predict performance measures. J. Biomech. **78**, 109–117 (2018)

100. M. White, N. Bezodis, J. Neville, H. Summers, Force-time curve alignment for functional principal component analysis in vertical jumping. ISBS - Conf. Proc. Arch. **38**(1), 320 (2020)

101. N.E. Helwig, S. Hong, E.T. Hsiao-Wecksler, J.D. Polk, Methods to temporally align gait cycle data. J. Biomech. **44**(3), 561–566 (2011)

102. Z. Geler, V. Kurbalija, M. Ivanović, M. Radovanović, W. Dai, Dynamic time warping: Itakura vs Sakoe-Chiba, in *2019 IEEE International Symposium on INnovations in Intelligent SysTems & Applications (INISTA)* (2019), pp. 1–6

103. J.O. Ramsay, Functional data analysis of juggling trajectories: rejoinder. Electron. J. Stat. **8**(2), 1874–1878 (2014)

104. CTW, Statistics of time warpings and phase variations (2012)

105. J.O. Ramsay, P. Gribble, S. Kurtek, Analysis of juggling data: Landmark and continuous registration of juggling trajectories. Electron. J. Stat. **8**(2), 1835–1841 (2014)

106. M. Bernardi, L.M. Sangalli, P. Secchi, S. Vantini, Analysis of proteomics data: Block k-mean alignment. Electron. J. Stat. **8**(2), 1714–1723 (2014)

107. X. Lu, J.S. Marron, Analysis of juggling data: object oriented data analysis of clustering in acceleration functions. Electron. J. Stat. **8**(2), 1842–1847 (2014)

108. S. Kurtek, Q. Xie, A. Srivastava, Analysis of juggling data: alignment, extraction, and modeling of juggling cycles. Electron. J. Stat. **8**(2), 1865–1873 (2014)

109. N.J.B. Brunel, J. Park, Removing phase variability to extract a mean shape for juggling trajectories. Electron. J. Stat. **8**(2), 1848–1855 (2014)

110. N.J.B. Brunel, J. Park, The Frenet-Serret framework for aligning geometric curves, in *Geometric Science of Information*, ed. by F. Nielsen, F. Barbaresco. Lecture Notes in Computer Science (Springer International Publishing, Cham, 2019), pp. 608–617

111. J. Wrobel, S.Y. Park, A.M. Staicu, J. Goldsmith, Interactive graphics for functional data analyses. Stat (Int. Stat. Inst.) **5**(1), 108–118 (2016)
112. M.G. Genton, Y. Sun, Functional data visualization, in *Wiley StatsRef: Statistics Reference Online* (American Cancer Society, New York, 2020), pp. 1–11
113. J. Tukey, *Exploratory Data Analysis*, 1st edn. (Pearson, London, 1977)
114. H. Wickham, L. Stryjewski, 40 years of boxplots. Technical Report, 2021
115. R.J. Hyndman, H.L. Shang, Rainbow plots, bagplots, and boxplots for functional data. J. Comput. Gr. Stat. **19**(1), 29–45 (2010)
116. S.López-Pintado, J. Romo, On the concept of depth for functional data. J. Am. Stat. Assoc. **104**(486), 718–734 (2009)
117. Y. Sun, M.G. Genton, Functional boxplots. J. Comput. Gr. Stat. **20**(2), 316–334 (2011)
118. J.O. Ramsay, S. Graves, G. Hooker, *fda: Functional data analysis* (2020). https://CRAN.R-project.org/package=fda. R package version 5.5.1
119. J. Wrobel, J. Goldsmith, *refund.shiny: Interactive Plotting for Functional Data Analyses* (2020). https://github.com/refunders/refund.shiny
120. L. Horváth, P. Kokoszka, Functional principal components, in *Inference for Functional Data with Applications*, ed. by L. Horváth, P. Kokoszka. Springer Series in Statistics (Springer, Berlin, 2012), pp. 37–43
121. C.M. Crainiceanu, A.M. Staicu, C.Z. Di, Generalized multilevel functional regression. J. Am. Stat. Assoc. **104**(488), 1550–1561 (2009)
122. K.J. Deluzio, U.P. Wyss, B.C.Y. Zee, P.A. Costigan, C. Sorbie, Principal component models of knee kinematics and kinetics: normal vs. pathological gait patterns. Hum. Mov. Sci. **16**(2–3), 201–217 (1997)
123. K.J. Deluzio, J.L. Astephen, Biomechanical features of gait waveform data associated with knee osteoarthritis: an application of principal component analysis. Gait Posture **25**(1), 86–93 (2007)
124. L. Xiao, Asymptotic properties of penalized splines for functional data. Bernoulli **26**(4), 2847–2875 (2020)
125. J.O. Ramsay, X. Wang, R. Flanagan, A functional data analysis of the pinch force of human fingers. J. R. Stat. Soc. C Appl. **44**(1), 17–30 (1995)
126. P. Hall, Principal component analysis for functional data: methodology, theory, and discussion, in *The Oxford Handbook of Functional Data Analysis*, ed. by F. Ferraty, Y. Romain (Oxford University Press, Oxford, 2010)
127. J.S. Morris, Comparison and contrast of two general functional regression modelling frameworks. Stat. Model. **17**, 59–85 (2017)
128. D. Backenroth, J. Goldsmith, M.D. Harran, J.C. Cortes, J.W. Krakauer, T. Kitago, Modeling motor learning using heteroscedastic functional principal components analysis. J. Am. Stat. Assoc. **113**(523), 1003–1015 (2018)
129. K. Davids, P. Glazier, D. Araújo, R. Bartlett, Movement systems as dynamical systems. Sports Med. **33**(4), 245–260 (2003)
130. M. Benko, W. Härdle, A. Kneip, Common functional principal components. Ann. Stat. **37**(1), 1–34 (2009)
131. B.N. Flury, Common principal components in K groups. J. Am. Stat. Assoc. **79**(388), 892–898 (1984)
132. M. Escabias, A.M. Aguilera, J.M. Heredia-Jiménez, E. Orantes-González, Functional data analysis in kinematics of children going to school, in *Functional Statistics and Related Fields*, ed. by G. Aneiros, G.E. Bongiorno, R. Cao, P.Vieu. Contributions to Statistics (Springer International Publishing, Cham, 2017), pp. 95–103
133. J. Cederbaum, M. Pouplier, P. Hoole, S. Greven, Functional linear mixed models for irregularly or sparsely sampled data. Stat. Model. **16**(1), 67–88 (2016)
134. M. Matabuena, M. Karas, S. Riazati, N. Caplan, P.R. Hayes, Estimating knee movement patterns of recreational runners across training sessions using multilevel functional regression models. Am. Stat. **77**(2), 169–181 (2023)

135. F. Scheipl, A.M. Staicu, S. Greven, Functional additive mixed models. J. Comput. Gr. Stat. **24**(2), 477–501 (2015)

136. F. Fan, J.T. Zhang, Two-step estimation of functional linear models with applications to longitudinal data. J. R. Stat. Soc. B Met. **62**(2), 303–322 (2000)

137. J.J. Faraway, Regression analysis for a functional response. Technometrics **39**(3), 254–261 (1997)

138. P.T. Reiss, L. Huang, M. Mennes, Fast function-on-scalar regression with penalized basis expansions. Int. J. Biostat. **6**(1) (2010)

139. S. Greven, F. Scheipl, A general framework for functional regression modelling. Stat. Model. **17**(1–2), 1–35 (2017)

140. S.N. Wood, *Generalized Additive Models: An Introduction with R*, 2nd edn. (Chapman & Hall/CRC, London, 2017)

141. S. Greven, F. Scheipl, Rejoinder. Stat. Model. **17**(1–2), 100–115 (2017)

142. J.S. Morris, V. Baladandayuthapani, R.C. Herrick, P. Sanna, H. Gutstein, Automated analysis of quantitative image data using isomorphic functional mixed models, with application to proteomics data. Ann. Appl. Stat. **5**(2A), 894–923 (2011)

143. R. Sergazinov, A. Leroux, E. Cui, C. Crainiceanu, R.N. Aurora, N.M. Punjabi, I. Gaynanova, A case study of glucose levels during sleep using multilevel fast function on scalar regression inference. Biometrics **79**(4), 3873–3882 (2023)

144. E. Cui, R. Li, C.M. Crainiceanu, L. Xiao, Fast multilevel functional principal component analysis. J. Comput. Gr. Stat. **32**(2), 366–377 (2023)

145. S. Greven, F. Scheipl, Comments on: inference and computation with generalized additive models and their extensions. TEST **29**(2), 343–350 (2020)

146. H. Zhu, P.J. Brown, J.S. Morris, Robust classification of functional and quantitative image data using functional mixed models. Biometrics **68**(4), 1260–1268 (2012)

147. B. Pietrosimone, M.K. Seeley, C. Johnston, S.J. Pfeiffer, J.T. Spang, J.T. Blackburn, Walking ground reaction force post-ACL reconstruction: Analysis of time and symptoms. Med. Sci. Sports Exerc. **51**(2), 246–254 (2019)

148. A.G.P. Andrade, J.C. Polese, L.A. Paolucci, H.J.K. Menzel, L.F. Teixeira-Salmela, Functional data analyses for the assessment of joint power profiles during gait of stroke subjects. J. Appl. Biomech. **30**(2), 348–352 (2014)

149. E. Passmore, H.K. Graham, M.G. Pandy, M. Sangeux, Hip- and patellofemoral-joint loading during gait are increased in children with idiopathic torsional deformities. Gait Posture **63**, 228–235 (2018)

150. H.C. Davis, B.A. Luc-Harkey, M.K. Seeley, J.T. Blackburn, B. Pietrosimone, Sagittal plane walking biomechanics in individuals with knee osteoarthritis after quadriceps strengthening. Osteoarthr. Cartil. **27**(5), 771–780 (2019)

151. S.J. Son, H. Kim, M.K. Seeley, J.T. Hopkins, Efficacy of sensory transcutaneous electrical nerve stimulation on perceived pain and gait patterns in individuals with experimental knee pain. Arch. Phys. Med. Rehabil. **98**(1), 25–35 (2017)

152. S.J. Son, H. Kim, M.K. Seeley, J.T. Hopkins, Movement strategies among groups of chronic ankle instability, coper, and control. Med. Sci. Sports Exerc. **49**(8), 1649–1661 (2017)

153. J. da SilvaSoares, F.P. Carpes, G. de FátimaGeraldo, F. BertúMedeiros, M. RobertoKunzler, Á. SosaMachado, L. AugustoPaolucci, A. Gustavo Pereirade Andrade, Functional data analysis reveals asymmetrical crank torque during cycling performed at different exercise intensities. J. Biomech. **122**, 110478 (2021)

154. G. Ramos DallaBernardina, M. Danillo Matosdos Santos, R. AlvesResende, M. Túliode Mello, M. RodriguesAlbuquerque, L. AugustoPaolucci, F.P. Carpes, A. Silva, A. Gustavo Pereirade Andrade, Asymmetric velocity profiles in Paralympic powerlifters performing at different exercise intensities are detected by functional data analysis. J. Biomech. **123**, 110523 (2021)

155. D. Nychka, Bayesian confidence intervals for smoothing splines. J. Am. Stat. Assoc. **83**(404), 1134–1143 (1988)

156. S.N. Wood, On confidence intervals for generalized additive models based on penalized regression splines. Aust. N.Z. J. Stat. **48**(4), 445–464 (2006)

157. T.C. Pataky, K. Abramowicz, D. Liebl, A. Pini, S.S. deLuna, L. Schelin, Simultaneous inference for functional data in sports biomechanics. AStA Adv. Stat. Anal. **107**, 369–392 (2021)

158. J.T. Zhang, ANOVA for functional data, in *Analysis of Variance for Functional Data* (Chapman & Hall/CRC, London, 2013)

159. Q. Shen, J. Faraway, An F test for linear models with functional responses. Stat. Sinica **14**(4), 1239–1257 (2004)

160. T. Górecki, L. Smaga, fdANOVA: an R software package for analysis of variance for univariate and multivariate functional data. Comput. Stat. **34**, 571–597 (2019)

161. T.C. Pataky, One-dimensional statistical parametric mapping in Python. Comput. Methods Biotech. Biomed. Eng. **15**(3), 295–301 (2012)

162. T.C. Pataky, Generalized n-dimensional biomechanical field analysis using statistical parametric mapping. J. Biomech. **43**(10), 1976–1982 (2010)

163. T.C. Pataky, rft1d: smooth one-dimensional random field upcrossing probabilities in Python. J. Stat. Softw. **71**, 1–22 (2016)

164. A. Pini, S. Vantini, The interval testing procedure: a general framework for inference in functional data analysis. Biometrics **72**(3), 835–845 (2016)

165. A. Pini, S. Vantini, Interval-wise testing for functional data. J. Nonparametr. Stat. **29**(2), 407–424 (2017)

166. G.M. James, J. Wang, J. Zhu, Functional linear regression that's interpretable. Ann. Stat. **37**(5A), 2083–2108 (2009)

167. P.T. Reiss, J. Goldsmith, H.L. Shang, R.T. Ogden, Methods for scalar-on-function regression. Int. Stat. Rev. **85**(2), 228–249 (2017)

168. B.X.W. Liew, D. Rugamer, A. Stocker, A.M. DeNunzio, Classifying neck pain status using scalar and functional biomechanical variables — development of a method using functional data boosting. Gait Posture **76**, 146–150 (2020)

169. B.X.W. Liew, D. Rugamer, A.M. DeNunzio, D. Falla, Interpretable machine learning models for classifying low back pain status using functional physiological variables. Eur. Spine J. **29**(8), 1845–1859 (2020)

170. S. Brockhaus, D. Rügamer, S. Greven, Boosting functional regression models with FDboost. J. Stat. Softw. **94**(1), 1–50 (2020)

171. N. Malfait, J.O. Ramsay, The historical functional linear model. Can. J. Stat. **31**(2), 115–128 (2003)

172. R Core Team, R: A Language and Environment for Statistical Computing, 2022

173. P. Kokoszka, M. Reimherr, Discussion of 'a general framework for functional regression modelling' by Greven and Scheipl. Stat. Model. **17**(1–2), 45–49 (2017)

174. C.M. Crainiceanu, A.M. Staicu, S. Ray, N. Punjabi, Bootstrap-based inference on the difference in the means of two correlated functional processes. Stat. Med. **31**(26), 3223–3240 (2012)

175. S.Y. Park, A.M. Staicu, L. Xiao, C.M. Crainiceanu, Simple fixed-effects inference for complex functional models. Biostat. **19**(2), 137–152 (2018)

176. E. Cui, A. Leroux, E. Smirnova, C.M. Crainiceanu, Fast univariate inference for longitudinal functional models. J. Comput. Graphical Stat. **31**(1), 219–230 (2022)

177. J. Goldsmith, T. Kitago, Assessing systematic effects of stroke on motorcontrol by using hierarchical function-on-scalar regression. J. R. Stat. Soc. C Appl. **65**(2), 215–236 (2016)

178. J.J. Faraway, *Extending the Linear Model with R : Generalized Linear, Mixed Effects and Nonparametric Regression Models* (Chapman & Hall/CRC, London, 2016)

179. J.S. Hodges, M.K. Clayton, Random effects old and new. *Richly Parameterized Linear Models: Additive, Time Series and Spatial Models Using Random Effects* (Chapman & Hall/CRC, 2013). https://api.semanticscholar.org/CorpusID:17938809

180. S. Greven, C.M. Crainiceanu, B. Caffo, D. Reich, Longitudinal functional principal component analysis. Electron. J. Stat. **4**, 1022–1054 (2010)

181. F. Abramovich, C. Angelini, Testing in mixed-effects FANOVA models. J. Stat. Plan. Inference **136**(12), 4326–4348 (2006)
182. A. Antoniadis, T. Sapatinas, Estimation and inference in functional mixed-effects models. Comput. Stat. Data Anal. **51**(10), 4793–4813 (2007)
183. A. Volkmann, A. Stöcker, F. Scheipl, S. Greven, Multivariate functional additive mixed models. Stat. Model. **23**(4), 303–326 (2021)
184. J.O. Ramsay, Differential equation models for statistical functions. Can. J. Stat. **28**(2), 225–240 (2000)
185. P.F. Lamb, R.M. Bartlett, Assessing movement coordination, in *Biomechanical Evaluation of Movement in Sport and Exercise*, 2nd edn. (Routledge, London, 2017)
186. J. Warmenhoven, S. Cobley, C. Draper, A.J. Harrison, N. Bargary, R. Smith, Bivariate functional principal components analysis: considerations for use with multivariate movement signatures in sports biomechanics. Sports Biomech. **18**(1), 10–27 (2019)
187. K.M. Trounson, A. Busch, N.F. Collier, S. Robertson, Effects of acute wearable resistance loading on overground running lower body kinematics. PLoS One **15**(12), e0244361 (2020)
188. A.J. Harrison, W. Ryan, K. Hayes, Functional data analysis of joint coordination in the development of vertical jump performance. Sports Biomech. **6**(2), 199–214 (2007)
189. I. Epifanio, C. Avila, A. Page, C. Atienza, Analysis of multiple waveforms by means of functional principal component analysis: normal versus pathological patterns in sit-to-stand movement. Med. Biol. Eng. Comput. **46**(6), 551–561 (2008)
190. K. Kipp, A.J. Cunanan, J. Warmenhoven, Bivariate functional principal component analysis of barbell trajectories during the snatch. Sports Biomech. **0**(0), 1–11 (2020)
191. S. Koner, A.M. Staicu, Second-generation functional data. Ann. Rev. Stat. Appl. **10**(1), 547–572 (2023)
192. J.O. Ramsay, Principal differential analysis: Data reduction by differential operators. J. R. Stat. Soc. B Met. **58**(3), 495–508 (1996)
193. J.O. Ramsay, Functional components of variation in handwriting. J. Am. Stat. Assoc. **95**(449), 9–15 (2000)
194. J.O. Ramsay, P. Gribble, Functional data analysis in action, in *Proceeding of the American Statistical Association* (1999)
195. P.F. Lamb, M. Stöckl, On the use of continuous relative phase: review of current approaches and outline for a new standard. Clin. Biomech. **29**(5), 484–493 (2014)
196. Y. Hurmuzlu, C. Basdogan, J.J. Carollo, Presenting joint kinematics of human locomotion using phase plane portraits and Poincaré maps. J. Biomech. **27**(12), 1495–1499 (1994)
197. A. Pini, J.L. Markström, L. Schelin, Test–retest reliability measures for curve data: an overview with recommendations and supplementary code. Sports Biomech. **0**(0), 1–22 (2019)
198. F.J.E. Telschow, M.R. Pierrynowski, S.F. Huckemann, Confidence tubes for curves on SO(3) and identification of subject-specific gait change after kneeling. J. R. Stat. Soc. C Appl. **72**(5), 1354–1374 (2023)
199. F.J.E. Telschow, M.R. Pierrynowski, S.F. Huckemann, Functional inference on rotational curves under sample-specific group actions and identification of human gait. Scand. J. Stat. **48**(4), 1256–1276 (2021)